Self-Help for Premenstrual Syndrome

Third Edition

Michelle Harrison, M.D.,

with Marla Ahlgrimm, R.Ph.

Self-Help
for
Premenstrual
Syndrome

Third Edition

Random House *New York*

The first edition of this work was published by Matrix Press, Cambridge,
Massachusetts, in 1982. The second edition was published by Random House, Inc., in 1985.

Library of Congress Cataloging-in-Publication Data

Harrison, Michelle.
Self-help for premenstrual syndrome / Michelle Harrison with Marla Ahlgrimm.—3rd ed.
p.   cm.
Includes bibliographical references and index.
ISBN 0-679-77800-4 (alk. paper)
1. Premenstrual syndrome. 2. Self-care, Health.   I. Ahlgrimm, Marla.   II. Title.
RG165.H37   1998
618.1′72—dc21   98-28036

Random House website address: www.atrandom.com
Printed in the United States of America

24689753

Third Edition

To Heather, Abigail, and Cecilia

Acknowledgments

❀

Each edition of this book has been shaped by the people, experiences, and challenges around me. I want to acknowledge those who forced me to think more, longer, and differently.

Drs. Michael Gallo and Robert Staab gave me a new understanding and respect for safety and quality control of biologically active agents. Drs. John Arbuthnott, Maureen Groer, Sobian Harlow, Sharon Hillier, Linda Lewis, Marian Melish, Zoltan Papp, Jeffrey Parsonnet, Raoul Reiser, James Roberts, Patrick Schlievert, and James Todd added to my understanding of the broad range of menstrual cycle effects on women's health. There were some colleagues whose seemingly simple questions forced me to think harder. Such was the case with Sir Gus Nossal, as I explored the relationship between menstruation and immunity. Digby Anderson helped me understand the links between public policy, junk science, and attitudes about health, as did Roger Bate with his rigorous scholarship in searching for truth in science. Dr. Lorraine Dennerstein moves comfortably across countries, continents, and cultures, and she broadened my understanding of menstrual attitudes around the world. So too did Dr. Nancy Reame with her work in China. Dr. Judith Esser-Mittag and I engaged in rich and ongoing discussions about the meaning of menstruation for young girls.

Barbara Seaman's questions, thoughts, and writing on women's health have challenged and guided me.

Dr. Carolyn Motzel upholds the core values of health education and opportunity in her global backyard.

Jack Mullen urged me to reach for the big ideas. He taught me to "think globally, and act globally too!"

Danny Strickland provided me with the opportunity to stretch, individually, and around the world. He taught me that what is heard is more important than what is said.

From my friends and colleagues Daryl Rand and Norman Vale, I learned more about global communications and about packaging thought, responsibly, so that it touches others, anyplace, anytime.

This revision could not have been completed without the long hours of work on the part of Treacy Colbert. She researched and mastered topic after topic that Marla and I requested, and always seemed to be right there at the other end of the E-mail at all hours of the day and night.

As always, Julie Popkin, my literary agent, offered ongoing support and encouragement.

I wish to thank Shirley and Joe Yetz for their warm support of me and my children in the creation of this book.

Writing can be hard on one's family. Mom may be right there, but still unavailable. I am grateful for the unqualified support and encouragement of my growing brood, Cici, Heather and Andrei, Shelley, Michael, and Lori.

Last, I am most indebted to my husband, Dr. James A. Wilson, for his love and friendship—and his editing. His patience and faith were an inspiration.

In the end, though, the opinions expressed are solely my own.

Preface to the Third Edition

The purpose of all health care is to allow people to go about their lives irrespective of how their bodies function. PMS, and the effects of the menstrual cycle on women's lives, had to be named. For what we do not name we cannot treat. What we do not treat lies hidden as vulnerability.

PMS and Women's Health

The recognition of PMS heralded a new era of women's health that began in the early 1980s and continues today. First came the tabloid reports of women who went on murderous rampages when they became premenstrual. In retrospect, we know that these women's problems were much more serious than PMS. However, the public attention to the cyclic changes of a woman's body at least validated what many women felt, namely, that their bodies and emotions differed (in nonmurderous ways) over the course of their menstrual cycles. This validation of their experiences empowered women and led them to speak out and to demand help.

A consumer-led movement began. Premenstrual-syndrome networks and information groups sprang up throughout the country. The media, although initially propelled by images of violent women with raging hormones, soon realized they had an even larger audience—healthy women who had some level of premenstrual discomfort, women with PMS. News reports became less sensational and began to focus on PMS as a women's health issue and then on women's health as a new and legitimate area for health consciousness. Because the only way to diagnose PMS was to "ask the patient," women became partners in their own diagnosis and medical care.

Medicine itself was undergoing a transformation. Research and treatment had been based upon the concept of a uniform medical population, which often omitted gender, age, race, and individual differences. Medicine was moving from a model of what works for *most* people to one that addressed more subtle differences among diverse populations. Research on women required consideration of the menstrual cycle because many conditions are affected by it. The menstrual phase can have a significant impact on drug dosage and effects, and medicine was beginning to realize this and integrate it into research and practice. A woman's menstrual cycle came to be seen not just as a monthly bleeding episode but as a constantly changing biological environment to be considered in all aspects of women's health.

PMS was just the beginning. A newly enlightened and educated population of women started to emerge. Women's health issues, which until then had been marginalized, entered the mainstream. The terms *PMS* and then *menopause,* previously relegated to whispers and "women only" groups, became part of everyday language. Women were hungry to understand their bodies and transcend its mysteries. And they did. The medical terminology of reproductive hormones became routine conversation.

A Historical Perspective

The current attention being paid to the effects of the menstrual cycle on women's health is not new, but the political environment in which it is being discussed is indeed different from that of the past. Historically, in Western culture, menstruation was indicative of weakness, of inferiority. Medical writings of the eighteenth century endorsed consideration of the menstrual cycle, but then only to argue that women were weaker, should not be educated, could not and should not take part in the leadership of society. In 1871 the president of the American Medical Association described woman as "unfitted by nature to become a physician." In the late nineteenth century a woman's functioning was not separated from that of her reproductive organs. Medical experts advocated removal of ovaries on the basis that "the moral sense of the patient is elevated. . . . She becomes tractable, orderly, industrious, and cleanly."

It was to be expected, given our history, that the question of reproductive hormones and behavior in women would become polarized and politicized. Recognizing biological differences and influences, without their becoming obstacles to women's opportunities, is the political and social challenge of our time. An individual woman may be empowered by the concept that hormones determine her feelings. But women, as a group, are disempowered by beliefs that their level of function is determined by their biology. This seeming contradiction must be considered when science is interpreted and used. In the meantime, we also have to identify and treat what, for individual women, may interfere in their achieving their own personal feeling of health, well-being, and success.

The Third Edition: Why Now?

For many years I have been asked when I would update this book. But until recently there didn't seem to be sufficient new research or information to warrant a new edition. The basic information in this book remains as valid today as it was when I wrote the first edition in 1981. It is based on the premise that women *do* know what they are feeling and that most PMS can be managed within the framework of self-help regimens.

But there is new information to be added and old and new myths to be dispelled.

- Interest and discussion about PMS has led to greater awareness and willingness to talk about menopause. (Perimenopause can be more about PMS than about menopause.)
- Recent studies demonstrate that women with PMS and women without PMS react differently to hormones, thus reinforcing a biological model of PMS.
- PMS is not mental illness, but some of the medications used for PMS are those used for depression and anxiety.
- The menstrual cycle can, at times, have an effect on other illnesses in women.
- Abundant resources are available on the Internet providing important information to keep you up to date.

This edition is written with the assistance of Marla Ahlgrimm, R.Ph., a pharmacist who was one of the pioneers in the recognition and treat-

ment of PMS. As founder and president of Women's Health America, she
continues to provide leadership to the medical community and to women
in identifying and understanding PMS and related conditions.

The Internet will increasingly provide information to all of us. One can
turn on a computer and find tens of thousands of references to PMS. Internet information is simple to obtain, and I encourage you to use it. A
book, however, is a framework. It places "self-help" in a context that includes learning about yourself, making some decisions, applying discipline—or choosing not to. A book should be a friend to return to again
and again as you put together what you feel with what you know, all in
the interest of moving your life toward greater fulfillment of your hopes
and aspirations.

Contents

❦

PART I

What Is PMS?

CHAPTER 1

❋

Introduction

How Do I Know That PMS Exists?

Medically, PMS is a striking phenomenon. In my medical practice, at lectures, and through the mail, thousands of women have told me such things as: "I'm not *me* that time of the month"; "My body swells up, and I look like I'm pregnant. My rings and shoes get tight"; "When I'm premenstrual the least little things make me cry"; "I just want to be alone and hide until I get my period"; "I can't go back to school because when I'm premenstrual I can't focus on the page"; "Getting my period is a bother, but being premenstrual is a nightmare."

As a child, I remember women sitting around a neighbor's kitchen table talking about irritability at *that time of month,* eating ice cream and potato chips at *that time of month,* and dealing with husbands and children at *that time of month.* They weren't talking about menstrual bleeding, for that had other expressions, like "having my friend" or "getting" it, said with a raising of one or both eyebrows that let everyone know what was meant.

It is clear that PMS exists, because among the thousands of women I have listened to, I have *never* had one say that each month, *after* her period, she loses self-esteem or fights with her husband or wants to kill herself. I've never heard a woman say that she wanted to feel *postmenstrually* as well as she does each month premenstrually. I've never heard a woman say, "You know, I get irritated easily, but premenstrually nothing could bother me." Whatever this phenomenon is, it appears to occur only pre-menstrually. Yes, women have difficulties at other times of the month, but those who have problems in relation to their menstrual cycles always re-port them as occurring premenstrually.

I'm struck by the diversity of the women I see: women in positions of power, who hold responsible jobs, but for whom PMS is a private agony; women living in poverty with three children still in diapers, who pre-menstrually struggle against their bodies and their living conditions to maintain a sense of order and hope. PMS has been reported around the world.

In 1982 I wrote of my feelings about PMS:

> *How do I feel about PMS? I am conflicted. The feminist in me wishes that our biology were irrelevant. The doctor in me sees the need for recognizing and treating premenstrual symptoms. The woman in me recognizes the power of the bi-ological forces within me and wishes I lived in a society in which my menstrual cycle was seen as an asset, not a liabil-ity. The writer in me keeps hoping that if you can get it all down on paper, you will not be alone in your dilemma or your conflict.*

It is possible that there are lessons for women *and* men in PMS. Is the greater sensitivity experienced by women premenstrually something we all, as a society, need to learn about? Without wanting to glorify or ro-manticize their pain, I wonder what growth will come to women as they confront PMS. What would the world be like if men sometimes seemed to cry without reason? What would we then believe about vulnerability or sensitivity?

Are there lessons to be learned from PMS regarding responsibility, anger, or violence, lessons applicable to both men and women? I wonder how we will look at PMS in twenty years. What will we have learned, and most important, how will we deal responsibly and compassionately with that knowledge?

Our strength as women must lie in our honesty and in our com-mitment to help each other, to concentrate on the ways we are more like each other than different. To these ends, we must continue to explore the cyclic nature of our lives, while remembering that our expressions and aspirations are still limited by a society in which we have not yet achieved equality.

This book examines the physical and emotional symptoms of PMS, their origins, and ways to deal with them. To provide this information, I have drawn on my work as a physician, on available research, and on traditional as well as nontraditional treatments found to be effective.

Much work remains to be done on PMS, and that process is well under way.

CHAPTER 2

❖

The PMS Dilemma

"You know you'll feel better when your period starts." Hours later, Alex's words still reverberated in Sally's head, making clear thought or action impossible. Behind the closed door of her office, she sat at her desk, twisting paper clips and crumpling tiny pieces of tissue paper.

In the minutes before leaving home that morning, Sally had said she was ending her marriage. She felt that she was at the end of caring, the end of giving, and had screamed at Alex that it was all over, that she wanted him to leave, that she couldn't stand living with him anymore. With a sinking feeling she realized that Amanda, their three-year-old, had heard the entire battle. She clutched the child and quickly left the house with her. Stopping briefly at the day-care center, she told the teachers that Amanda might be upset and then guiltily went on to work.

Driving along the river, gliding in and out of slow and faster lanes, she experienced confusion, despair, and anger. She wasn't sure who she was, what she was feeling, or why. The driving helped her, creating the distance she needed now in her struggle for inner clarity.

Mornings were always the worst, when she woke to find herself between the fading darkness and dreams. Sally needed to be alone when she awakened, to gather slowly the strength for the demands that seemed to drain her. That need seemed especially strong this morning. She had awakened feeling bloated, wanting to hold on to the darkness that hid the distortions of her body, kept her from the mirror and skirt snaps that were the enemies of her self-esteem. Her skin had crawled, and she had thought that if only the world would leave her alone, she might just make it through.

Work was a different world. Here, where she managed the production department of a major trade publication, she competently made decisions, negotiated, managed people and policies. Here her life with Alex seemed unreal. Shuffling papers, trying to overcome her despair, she fought the intruding thought: Was her marriage over?

Had Alex been right? That question, one she sometimes asked herself and sometimes fled, now left her feeling sick, vulnerable, and naked. *If this were a week from now, would she feel better?* After her period arrived, would she simply smile and say she must have been tired? Would the rage, confusion, and desperate need to be alone have vanished?

Does Sally have *premenstrual syndrome*? Will she be all right when her period starts? Which is the "real" Sally? Is she out of control premenstrually, or is she simply suppressing her real feelings the rest of the month? Does Sally have an illness, as is implied by the word *syndrome,* or is she experiencing the mood shifts that are a normal part of everyone's life?

What about other women? What about women who have a day of blues premenstrually? What about women who are premenstrually suicidal or unable to function? Are those states all separate conditions, or are they points on a continuum, and at what point is it "illness"?

In the past fifty years we have seen the increased medicalization of women's normal functions. Childbirth has become a technological event, often a surgical procedure. Menopause is often seen as a disease to be treated, frequently in the face of the woman's protest that she feels fine and doesn't need or want medication.

In looking at illness, Western culture traditionally tends to split the body from the mind, to see the two as distinct entities, often unrelated. If we define a disease as physical, then we are not responsible for it. If it is emotional, then we not only assign blame for its development (parents have done it to us, et cetera) but are also held responsible for overcoming it. We tend to believe that physical disease happens to us and that mental disease we bring on ourselves.

In recent years medicine has given more attention to the intricate interplay between body and mind. Heart disease and cancer are physical diseases that have been shown to be strongly influenced by environment, diet, stress, and personality dynamics. Depression, an emotional disorder, also has physical manifestations, including at times biochemical changes now measurable with laboratory testing. Whether the biochemical change is a cause or a result of the depression remains unanswered. Women living together in dormitories unknowingly begin to synchronize their menstrual cycles. Testosterone levels in males are altered by their positions of dominance. Hormones can produce emotional changes. And social interactions can elicit hormonal changes.

Premenstrual syndrome is usually described as a disorder either of body (advocates of that theory believe there is a basic biological flaw in a large percentage of women of reproductive age) or of mind (a woman with PMS has not "accepted her role as a woman"). The issue of whether PMS is physical or mental becomes further polarized because of the significance we place on whether we can define an illness as physical or emotional. But in fact, all diseases raise this issue. PMS is just one more example.

Physicians said for years that dysmenorrhea, severe menstrual cramps, were due to a woman's ambivalence about womanhood. When prostaglandins were discovered to be related to the cramping, this theory lost favor, but in the meantime generations of women were treated as though this belief were fact. Women were told they had cramps because they didn't like being women, that they were "rejecting the feminine role."

Our culture has a negative attitude toward menstruation. Little notice has been made of women who report increased efficiency, creativity, and sensitivity during their premenstrual times, sometimes even in the presence of uncomfortable physical or emotional states. Professionals often have difficulty hearing what women are really saying, and thus even the research can be tainted by personal biases. For example, attempts are made to separate what women "really" feel from what they "think" they feel, a distinction that implies an inability to hear what is being said and an assumption that there is a difference between the two.

The situation continues to improve. The dramatic changes in women's health over the past twenty years have mostly been in the willingness of the health care community to take seriously the concerns of women. Women's health care services abound, as do books and information. Women have options today, for information and for care.

CHAPTER 3

❋

The Many Symptoms of PMS

A LL THE SYMPTOMS OF PMS can occur as part of other illnesses or other life experiences. What characterizes them as PMS is their *cyclicity*—their persistent, repetitive occurrence on a monthly basis prior to menstruation. Having one or even a few of these symptoms does not necessarily mean that you are ill, but being incapacitated by them does. Thoughts and actions are not the same.

> *Approximately fifteen days after the start of my monthly period I find myself with complete lack of interest in life in general. I have problems with vision and craving for food. I become anxious, lose interest in sex. This started three years ago and became gradually worse with time. After fourteen days I am back to normal. My doctor calls it nerves, but when I ask him why it lasts fourteen days and hits me at the same time every month, he shakes his head and leaves the room. One of his thoughts is that most women need more sex.*
>
> *My husband is so sensitive to my feelings he will say to me, "It started again. I can tell by the expression on your face. You don't have to hide it. I only wish I could help."*

Any of the following symptoms may occur premenstrually as part of PMS:

abdominal bloating	*irritability*
abdominal cramping	*joint swelling and pain*
absentmindedness	*lack of coordination*
accident-proneness	*lactation difficulties*
acne	*lethargy*
alcohol intolerance	*muscle aches*
anger	*nausea*
anxiety	*noise sensitivity*
asthma	*palpitations (heart pounding)*
back pain	*panic*
breast swelling and pain	*paranoia*
cardiac arrhythmia (irregular heartbeat)	*pimples*
confusion	*rashes*
cravings for sweets	*salt cravings*
crying	*seizures*
depression	*self-esteem loss*
dizziness	*sex-drive changes*
eating disorders	*slurred speech*
edema	*smell sensitivity*
eye difficulties	*spaciness*
fainting	*stiff neck*
fatigue	*styes*
food binges	*suicidal thoughts*
hand tingling and numbness	*tension*
headaches	*tiredness*
hemorrhoids (flare-ups)	*touch sensitivity*
herpes (oral, skin, genital)	*urinary difficulties*
hives	*violence*
indecisiveness	*weight gain*
infections	*withdrawal*
insomnia	

The Cycle Is the Link

The actual symptoms of PMS in this list are generally considered nonspecific—that is, they are not indicative of any one cause but may result from many different disorders. For instance, allergy, hypoglycemia (low blood sugar), chemical toxins, tension, brain tumors, stress, or nutritional disorders may cause headache. Anemia, stress, or a vitamin deficiency may cause fatigue. The *timing* of the symptoms determines whether a woman has PMS. For example, the fatigue of PMS occurs *only* premenstrually. If fatigue is caused by anemia, a woman will feel fatigued all month. Generally, premenstrual symptoms begin sometime after ovulation and end with menstruation.

Characteristics of PMS Symptoms

· They begin sometime between ovulation and menstruation.
· They range from mild and hardly noticeable to severe and incapacitating.
· They disappear, often abruptly, each month with the onset of menses or shortly thereafter.
· They last anywhere from one or two days to two weeks.
· They may occur at any time in a woman's life, from menarche (the first menstrual period) to past menopause.
· They tend to become more severe with age.
· They may be attributed to early menopause or perimenopause but may actually be PMS that has become more severe with age.
· They may occur after a hysterectomy, with or without removal of ovaries.
· They may occur after tubal ligation or even after tubal or ovarian surgery.
· They may occur after several illnesses or major physical, emotional, or sexual traumas.
· They may occur some months and not others.
· They may be more severe some months than others.
· They are usually somewhat consistent but at times may vary from month to month.

How the Physical Symptoms Are Experienced

ABDOMINAL BLOATING, JOINT SWELLING, EDEMA (GENERALIZED WATER RETENTION):

> *I feel as if I have gained a hundred pounds, and I can barely tolerate my children. I feel as if I am going to jump out of my skin.*

Nothing fits, and I sometimes think that if I stuck a pin in my body, all this water would pour out.

Premenstrually, water may collect in the tissues of the abdomen as well as in the ankles and other joints and in the face. Although some women do gain weight during this time (as much as ten to twelve pounds each month), body fluids are being redistributed. Some women experience an increase in thirst. Others have a characteristic puffiness around their eyes. Some models and actresses try to avoid having photographs taken at that time because of the change in their appearance. You may need to wear larger clothes premenstrually because of abdominal bloating. Many women complain that they have to keep two sizes of clothing to wear at different times in their cycles. Your shoes may feel tight, and if you are dieting, you may get discouraged because of the bloating or weight gain. Typically this excess water disappears around the first day of the menstrual period.

ABDOMINAL CRAMPING:

Two weeks prior to menstruation I begin to experience pain, swelling, and exhaustion. By two days before menstruation I have cramping. And terrible cramps, nausea, and weakness come with the start of menstruation. I do not suffer from depression or mood swings.

My abdomen feels tender, especially if I sit down fast.

It's a feeling of a pull that goes from my vagina down both thighs.

Premenstrual cramps, which can feel a lot like menstrual cramps, can occur up to two weeks before the period begins. They may or may not be followed by heavy menstrual cramps. Often the cramping begins at midcycle, the time of ovulation, and either continues full force or else abates until just before the period begins. Cramping may also be felt in the back, thighs, or vaginal area.

ACCIDENT-PRONENESS, LACK OF COORDINATION, SLURRED SPEECH:

I know I'm premenstrual when I start cutting my fingers slicing vegetables.

One of the more subtle but troublesome symptoms of PMS is the decrease in physical coordination that can result in women tripping more easily, dropping things, feeling less able to carry out usually easy physical tasks. Some athletes and dancers say that their timing is off. Singers may find their voices altered, not as fine, and may dread performances premenstrually.

ACNE, HIVES, STYES, PIMPLES, RASHES:

> *When am I going to outgrow adolescence? I always have blackheads but get a fresh crop of pimples monthly, and it takes nearly a month to get them to clear up.*

Acne is not *caused* by PMS, but many women, adult and teen, find that their acne becomes much worse premenstrually. Women who don't usually have skin problems may break out with pimples or sores at this time of month. If a woman is prone to styes or other infections, including herpes, these problems may erupt premenstrually. Some women are more allergic to makeup; others report that their makeup doesn't look right at this time of month.

ALCOHOL INTOLERANCE:

> *I became an alcoholic due to PMS because I found that if I lived like a zombie I wouldn't feel anything.*

> *My doctor told me a glass of wine might make me relax at night.*

Perhaps you don't usually notice any effects from four ounces of wine or a glass of beer, but premenstrually you may feel as though you've had several times that amount. Furthermore, some women resort to alcohol as a solution to premenstrual mood changes and physical discomforts. (I do not recommend this.) There is therefore a clear-cut relationship between alcoholism and PMS. The combination of increased sensitivity to alcohol premenstrually and alcohol's depressing effect result in a self-perpetuating pattern of alcohol consumption and depression.

ASTHMA: Asthma is certainly not caused by PMS, but there are women whose asthma occurs primarily premenstrually. This may or may not be in association with generalized increased infections and allergic reactions.

Asthma is a condition that can be affected by infection, allergy, stress, and emotions.

BACK PAIN, JOINT PAIN, MUSCLE ACHES, STIFF NECK: Few people chart their aches and pains in relation to their menstrual cycles. Orthopedists are becoming increasingly aware, however, that unexplained recurrent pain in the back and other muscles may be related to a woman's cycle. Commonly the pains begin in one area, as with a stiff neck, and over the course of a week or so tend to travel to the back or legs. Traditionally these pains have simply been ignored as "women's complaints."

BREAST SWELLING AND PAIN:

> *I can't stand the sheet touching my breasts.*

> *The breast pain begins between one to two weeks before the onset of my period. The consistency of my breasts changes when the pain begins. They usually feel mildly lumpy, but premenstrually they become quite hard near my underarms and many small tube-shaped lumps can be felt around the outside of each breast. The lumps are very tender and hurt when touched. My breasts at this time feel extremely heavy and sore all over. Under my arms and on the part of my breast closest to my underarms I feel extremely sharp pains. Sometimes I feel the pain all the way down my arm. It is usually greatest in the morning and at night. This breast pain lasts from one to two weeks before my period until two to three days after my period has started.*

The breast symptoms that occur with PMS can be mild or quite severe. The swelling and soreness can result in extreme sensitivity to any touch, including clothing. Breast cysts tend to become enlarged at this time, and women whose breast tissue is usually smooth may develop lumps. These symptoms usually disappear within a few days of the onset of the period.

CONFUSION, ABSENTMINDEDNESS, SPACINESS, INDECISIVENESS:

> *It's like a thin wall of glass is set up in my head.*

> *I've had some of my best moments in the courtroom even though I've felt premenstrually spacey inside. I can't explain*

it. I dread those days because of how I feel, but I always seem to come through. Sometimes I think I'm just going on automatic pilot.

Memory difficulties or a vague sense of "not thinking quite right" can occur premenstrually. Strangely, other people may have no idea that a woman is having this difficulty. These are intriguing symptoms because some extremely competent and highly functioning women report having them. They say that because of the pressure of their work they can overcome them. Unfortunately, others are severely incapacitated by these problems.

CRAVINGS FOR SWEETS AND/OR SALT: The physiological changes in a woman's body premenstrually often result in hunger and specific food cravings. The most common foods craved are chocolate and salty chips. This is the most difficult time for dieting women because they find it hardest to refrain from sweets and often become discouraged because of their binges. Women caught in the cycle of anorexia, bingeing, and self-induced vomiting often have their most difficult times premenstrually. Liking chocolate per se is not a symptom of PMS, but going out at midnight in a rainstorm to get it is indicative of having—and giving in to—a strong craving. Doing this repeatedly shortly before you get your period is symptomatic of a premenstrual craving. If this behavior significantly interferes with your life, you have PMS.

EATING DISORDERS, ANOREXIA, BULIMIA:

I know it seems like an exaggeration, but it's as though a hungry monster inside me were ready to devour anything sweet, especially chocolate. I'll stuff and stuff myself. Then after I'm done, I'm suddenly calm. I can't believe I lost control again. Sometimes I make myself throw up; sometimes I am just depressed and don't bother.

I have been a borderline anorexic for years. Premenstrually though, all I can think about is food. I stare at it, count calories in volume, imagine eating it. I rarely actually give in to bingeing, but it's hard not to.

We are living at a time when there is an epidemic of eating disorders among women. PMS greatly exacerbates these, partly because of the food cravings and changes in appetite. Women get into a pattern of bingeing premenstrually, followed by laxative use or self-induced vomiting or by starvation between binges and after the period begins.

EYE DIFFICULTIES:

>   *I can't read for fourteen days.*

Regularly recurring eye problems can include excessive dryness, tearing (to be differentiated from crying), difficulty focusing, and aching.

FAINTING AND DIZZINESS: Sometimes in the absence of any diagnosed medical condition, women will experience these symptoms premenstrually.

FATIGUE, LETHARGY, TIREDNESS:

>   *I think on those days that I'll never be able to move again. I mean, I really think that this is the end, that my body has quit on me.*

Women can experience fatigue throughout the premenstrual time or, more commonly, one or two days prior to the onset of menstruation. This pervasive sense of exhaustion can occur without any of the mood changes.

HAND TINGLING AND NUMBNESS: These can occur, only premenstrually, without any evidence of known neurological diseases that could account for them.

HEADACHES: All types of headaches, including migraines and tension headaches, can occur more frequently or solely during the premenstrual time for women with PMS. Often the migraines occur on the day before the period or during the first two days of bleeding. Some women have headaches starting shortly *after* their periods begin. This is not PMS, but it is a menstrually related phenomenon that is now being recognized because women have begun keeping track of when their headaches occur.

HEMORRHOIDS: Hemorrhoids are not caused by PMS, but they can be much more troublesome during that phase of the cycle. They tend to hurt more and they bleed more.

INFECTIONS: Many infections seem to occur on a regular basis premenstrually. These include sinus infections, sore throat, herpes (cold sores and genital herpes), skin boils, urinary-tract infections, and others. These infections are caused by the usual organisms, but there seems to be a decrease in the body's resistance at this time and therefore an exacerbation of symptoms.

INSOMNIA: Premenstrual sleeplessness can occur independent of any mood changes and in women who otherwise sleep well. In fact, the insomnia often begins before other symptoms and may contribute to mood shifts, irritability, and depression. The insomnia can consist either of difficulty falling asleep at night or of awakening too early in the morning.

LACTATION DIFFICULTIES: Contrary to popular belief, women often menstruate while they are still nursing. Premenstrually they may find changes both in quality and quantity of the milk. Babies may react differently to nursing in the few days before menstruation. These changes are somewhat more frequent among women who are relactating or attempting to lactate in order to nurse an adopted baby.

MENSTRUAL CRAMPS (DYSMENORRHEA): These are *not* part of PMS. In fact, women with PMS more often have painless periods, though some do have both PMS and severe menstrual cramping. Women with PMS tend to look forward to getting their periods because of the relief they feel, even in the presence of cramps; women with dysmenorrhea more often dread their periods. The presence of menstrual cramps is *not* an indication of PMS.

NAUSEA: This occurs often in conjunction with dizziness and premenstrual cramping.

PALPITATIONS (HEART POUNDING), CARDIAC ARRHYTHMIA (IRREGULAR HEARTBEAT):

> *I have anxious feelings with skin tingling; I have been hospitalized five times for heart palpitations. I've been to many doctors, and they haven't found a cause for the palpitations.*

Cardiac irregularities can be an indication of serious and potentially dangerous cardiac conditions. Often, especially when they occur only premenstrually, a cause is not found, but they should always be thoroughly investigated.

SEIZURES:

> *My seizures come premenstrually even though they are treated with medication. I get scared and forget where I am, and then I cry easily.*

Some women with seizure disorders find that their seizures are more common premenstrually. This is true of grand mal, petit mal, and temporal-lobe seizures.

SENSITIVITY TO NOISE, TOUCH, SMELL:

> *Two weeks after my period, my breasts swell, my joints ache, and I feel lower-back pain. Then one week later it's depression, sensitivity to loud noise, and general sense of loss of control.*

> *When I say to my mother, "That smells terrible," she says, "You must be getting your period."*

> *I don't want to be touched.*

> *I can't wear wool premenstrually.*

> *My jewelry begins to irritate me premenstrually.*

Women most often report an increased sensitivity to touch and hearing, but some also react strongly to certain smells. The sensitivity to sound ranges from being more bothered by a baby's crying to finding the radio or TV much too loud. The sensitivity to touch includes specific tender areas of the body as well as a generalized sensation of discomfort when the skin is touched.

SEX-DRIVE CHANGES:

> *One day of extreme fatigue every month—I could spend that day in bed. Despite extreme fatigue I experience hypersexuality, sexual thoughts, and a feeling of just barely keeping my sex drive under control.*

> *My husband and I have a good sex life, but premenstrually I couldn't care less and I know it hurts him to have me feel that way.*

These changes in sex drive will be described more fully in Chapter 19. Both increased and decreased libido can occur during the premenstrual phase.

URINARY DIFFICULTIES: Increased frequency of urination and burning on urination can occur premenstrually even in the absence of known infection. Some women seem to have an increase in the sensitivity of the urinary tract as well as of the vaginal area.

WEIGHT GAIN: Some women feel as though they have gained weight even though the scale does not show an increase. Others have reported as much as a twelve-pound weight gain and loss monthly because of fluid retention. The weight gain of PMS is complicated by edema, food cravings, and binges.

Emotional Symptoms

ANGER, ANXIETY, CRYING, DEPRESSION, IRRITABILITY, LOSS OF SELF-ESTEEM, PANIC, PARANOIA, SUICIDAL THOUGHTS, TENSION, VIOLENCE, WITHDRAWAL: The emotional symptoms, more than any others, bring women to seek help for PMS. In my first year of treating women with PMS, I was consulted by a woman of limited means from Nevada who had traveled to Boston at great financial hardship. When I asked her why she had come, she answered, slowly, "Well, each month my breasts hurt and my abdomen swells up . . ." She paused. Few women travel across the country for bloating and breast tenderness. "And," she continued, staring at the floor, "I'm a bitch."

She was describing PMS.

> *Just about a week before my periods I begin to go into a world of like a mental illness—crying jags, phobias about going outside, like impending doom—constantly thinking about dying. I am not a suicidal person, but I need help in this area.*

> *I become so snappish I have to keep myself from firing people on my staff.*

> *I feel as if I'm in a dark hole and can't get out.*

Obviously, all these emotions are common to both men and women and can occur at all times of the month. It is their *cyclic* and often unexplained presence premenstrually that characterizes them as premenstrual syndrome.

Women frequently seek help for PMS because of the emotional costs and pain to their families, friends, and coworkers. They are often more worried about the effects of their PMS on others than on themselves. Women with children frequently seek help because they fear losing control around the children or hurting them as a result of their unpredictable mood changes.

> *I have a feeling of hatred toward others, and I withdraw*
> *so I won't hurt anyone.*

Some women experience what feels to them like a complete personality change, as though an outside force had just replaced Dr. Jekyll with Mr. Hyde. This change often includes feelings of anger, loss of control, and despair, most of which disappear with the onset of menstruation. The woman is left with a memory of having been someone other than her present self, and with guilt for emotions expressed and actions taken during that time.

> *I'd even be okay if I knew I'd always be premenstrual.*
> *Even while I'm angry with my husband I know I will change*
> *and regret what I am saying. If I could be angry consistently,*
> *I'd be better. It's the change that's so difficult.*

The change is unpredictable and often takes place without warning. It can be a matter of waking up one morning feeling tense, angry, irritable, knowing that anything anyone says will seem wrong, that anything that doesn't go as planned will result in anger or tears beyond what the reality of the situation would warrant. An attorney who premenstrually is experiencing sadness might lose a case and then believe that to be the cause of her sadness, when on another day she would take the same loss in stride. If she is feeling angry and someone says something that annoys her, a woman may react out of proportion and even assume that what was said or done is the cause of her feeling. People around her are often left with the sense that they can't do anything right.

I know I'm premenstrual when I'm driving along and suddenly I find myself calling other drivers assholes! I never use that word at any other time.

Some mornings I just feel this terrible anger in me. I'm climbing the walls, and I think I pick a fight with my husband just for the release of the tension. I tell myself I have reason to be angry at the time, but I know inside I need to fight with him.

For many women, however, the personality change is not so complete, nor are the issues so unrelated to reality as they would like to believe. Our society discourages the expression of anger by women, and during the premenstrual period those feelings may be less easily held in check. Many women have said that this is the one time when they can say whatever is on their minds.

Often the issues over which a woman is upset premenstrually are real ones, but at this time she is unable to express them constructively. Once the "loss of control" has passed, the woman, filled with guilt for how she expressed herself, looks back and says, "Oh, it really isn't important. I was just premenstrual." Those around her tend also to dismiss her complaints with "Oh, she was just being premenstrual." The validity of her concerns is thus denied both by the woman and by others. She feels guilty for her reaction, brushes it off, and like the perpetual dieter, promises herself that it won't happen again.

As I began to understand my PMS, I saw that I had been like a pot with a heavy lid. When I wasn't premenstrual and something was on my mind, I just stuck it in the pot and forgot about it. But then when I was premenstrual it was as though the lid was loosened and all the stuff I'd been burying came blasting out at everyone, including me.

Being in Control

For many women, being in control at all times is basic to their functioning and sense of stability. Physiological changes that lessen control of their emotions can threaten their self-esteem, identity, and sense of femininity.

Few women actually lose control, but the feeling that it is about to be lost can be terrifying.

Women tend to be defensive about their premenstrual experiences. One woman described her despair about PMS like this: "I'm a graphic artist, but for two weeks out of the month I'm worthless at work. I just can't do as well as I can the rest of the time." Asked about her general performance, whether she thought she contributed as much to her job as the men in her office, she quickly and easily responded, "Oh, yes, I'm certainly as good as they are. I'm actually the best person in the department." Asked if sometimes the men perform at less than their full potential, she said, "Sure, every time something goes wrong at home or in business, they're useless at work too. It happens to them all the time." Women often hold themselves to a standard of performance that on a sustained basis is unrealistic for anyone.

Heightened Consciousness

PMS in some ways resembles an altered state of consciousness, an experience of being in a different world, of looking at life through a magnifying lens. It is often a world with its own internal consistency. Some women describe an enhancement of creativity and perceptiveness, a richness of sensation and imagery lacking at other times.

A sculptor described her special abilities when she was premenstrual.

> There is a quality to my work and to my vision that just isn't there the rest of the month. I look forward to being premenstrual for its effect on my creativity, although some of the other symptoms create strains with my family.

Another woman, prone to depression, described the journal she kept:

> When I am premenstrual I can write with such clarity and depth that after I get my period I don't recognize that those were my thoughts or that I could have written anything so profound.

An aide in a nursing home reported that when she was premenstrual she became upset about the treatment of the patients. When she saw the old people neglected and suffering, she was more empathic and often broke down in tears. When she was premenstrual, she harbored fantasies of calling the health department to close the place. When she was not premenstrual, she still did not like what she saw, but she would become more "realistic" and able to cope with the situation.

CHAPTER 4

❀

Causes of PMS

A WOMAN WITH PMS IS basically healthy; each physiological process works well for *part of each month.* Most of the time the woman's body knows how to excrete water and salt efficiently. Most of the time women with PMS have normal moods—with normal ups and downs. Their basic reproductive functioning is normal—they usually do ovulate, do conceive, and do carry to term. Basically everything works, but sometimes not as well as it could.

PMS represents a physiological change of the body's regulatory and modulating mechanisms. Signals are crossed, lost, or distorted but only some of the time. It is as though the body were an orchestra. Each instrument or set of instruments is able to play well, but then, for *part of the month,* something goes wrong with how the orchestra is conducted.

Where Is the Conductor?

The hypothalamus is the regulatory center of the body. It is an area in the center of the brain where the neurological and endocrine systems are integrated. The hypothalamus receives nerve and hormonal input from the other parts of the brain and from the rest of the body; then it sends out messages controlling the nervous and endocrine functions of the body. It is likely that the hypothalamus is the conductor that, in PMS, goes awry during part of the menstrual cycle.

The hypothalamus is involved, either directly or indirectly, in the following bodily processes:

• It secretes hormones and stimulates the anterior pituitary gland. This gland in turn affects the following:

  · breasts—stimulation of milk production directly and breast-tissue fullness indirectly.
  · thyroid gland—control of basic metabolic functioning of cells.
  · adrenal glands—steroid production and partial blood-glucose control.
  · ovaries—hormones from the pituitary gland stimulate development of cells that lead to ovulation and to estrogen and progesterone production. These hormones also affect libido.
  · tissue and bone growth through the secretion of growth hormone.

• It stimulates the posterior pituitary gland, whose hormones affect uterine contractions and labor as well as water and electrolyte balance.
• It directly stimulates portions of the autonomic nervous system, thereby affecting:

  · heart rate.
  · blood pressure.
  · heat regulation through shivering, panting, sweating.
  · gastrointestinal movement and glucose-level regulation.
  · constriction and relaxation of bronchial tubes in the lungs.

Specific centers within the hypothalamus also regulate more specific functions, many of which seem to operate poorly premenstrually.

• A thermoregulatory center adjusts the body to maintain body temperature.
• An appetite center registers both hunger and satisfaction, thus influencing eating behavior.
• A weight-control center seems to "set" body weight.
• Specific emotional centers in the hypothalamus are poorly understood, but animal studies have demonstrated that:

· stimulation of some centers produces responses suggestive of reward and punishment.

· stimulation of punishment centers results in a pattern of behavior called "rage" because the animal responds as if to attack.

· stimulation of some areas causes reactions that seem to be anxiety and fear.

• Susceptibility to rage seems to follow destruction of some parts of the hypothalamus in humans.

When you look at the long list of PMS symptoms in the previous chapter, you can see how many of them can be seen as being related to hypothalamic functioning.

What Affects the Hypothalamus?

The hypothalamus operates by *feedback*—that is, by responding to what is already happening in the body. If the temperature is too high or too low, it directs the appropriate changes in activity—sweating or shivering—to bring the temperature back within normal range. This kind of subtle shifting is occurring all the time in response to physical conditions as well as to levels of circulating hormones.

The hypothalamus also responds to chemicals secreted by nerve endings. These substances, called neurotransmitters, can affect mood. One neurotransmitter, serotonin, has been implicated in depression. The hypothalamus is bathed in these neurotransmitters, which in turn stimulate hypothalamic activity and hormone production or even become transformed into hormones themselves. Exposure to light can influence hypothalamic function and the amount of hormone production. It is sensitive to day/night cycles as well as to monthly ones.

The hypothalamus is directly connected to other parts of the brain and receives stimulation from them. For instance, certain nerve fibers connect olfactory (smell) centers with the hypothalamus, so stimulation by smell can affect the hypothalamus. In this system, stress and mood can *themselves* result in hormonal changes.

Heredity, trauma, nutrition (including hormones ingested in foods and food supplements), infection, and many yet-to-be-determined factors can also influence hypothalamic functioning.

Why the hypothalamus does not function well for part of the month is not known. Nevertheless, pieces of the puzzle are beginning to be understood, most of them related to parts of individual systems affected. To return to the analogy of the orchestra, we are beginning to find what is wrong with some of the players premenstrually as well as to understand more about what influences the conductor's control of the orchestra.

The Menstrual Cycle

The menstrual cycle is the clearest demonstration of the cyclicity of a woman's hormonal function. It results from an interplay of the hypothalamus, pituitary gland, and ovaries, through elaborate feedback mechanisms. The rise and fall of hormones governing the menstrual cycle happens over and over again, an intricate pattern repeating itself in remarkably consistent fashion each month.

The cycle is divided into two phases of approximately fourteen days each. (The twenty-eight-day cycle is used as an average—women's cycles vary from twenty-two to thirty-five or more days.)

The first half of the cycle is called the *follicular* phase. It starts on Day 1, when menstruation begins, and lasts approximately until Day 14, just before ovulation occurs.

On Day 1, the lining of the uterus begins to slough as a period—there is no fertilized egg. Estrogen and progesterone levels are low. As the follicular phase continues, estrogen begins to rise, stimulating the growth of the uterine lining. Progesterone remains low during this half of the cycle.

Prompted by the "conductor" (hypothalamus), the pituitary gland in the brain signals the ovaries to produce follicle-stimulating hormone (FSH). FSH stimulates a follicle (egg) in the ovary to mature or ripen.

At midcycle, estrogen reaches its highest level. This estrogen surge or peak stimulates the release of luteinizing hormone (LH) from the brain. LH prompts the ripened follicle to be released from the ovary (ovulation). Some women feel a cramping or pinching sensation on one side when they ovulate—this is called mittelschmerz. There may also be some midcycle spotting or bleeding. Estrogen drops sharply as the egg is released.

Ovulation marks the end of the follicular phase and the beginning of the second half of the menstrual cycle, or *luteal* phase. During the luteal phase, the (now empty) follicle becomes the *corpus luteum* (meaning "yellow body," describing the appearance of the egg).

After ovulation, the level of progesterone begins to rise in the body, peaking at around Day 21. If the egg has been fertilized by sperm, progesterone will continue to rise. If pregnancy hasn't occurred, the egg disintegrates. Progesterone begins to drop, continuing to decline until Day 28. This drop-off in progesterone triggers the lining of the uterus to be shed as a period roughly fourteen days after ovulation. The cycle begins all over again.

PMS symptoms occur in the second half, or luteal phase. For some women, symptoms begin at ovulation and last for a full two weeks. Other women experience symptoms for only a few days before their period starts. Premenstrual symptoms end at about the same time menstrual bleeding begins.

What Does Not Cause PMS

While we do not know what causes PMS, we do know what does *not* cause it.

PMS seems to occur in many different cultures around the world. However, the specific symptoms tend to vary. In some parts of the world the symptoms are more physical. Most of what has been written about the cycle has been about menstruation itself rather than about PMS. And much of this literature has been clouded by the stigma attached to menstruation.

Because PMS is so elusive and confusing, there is a tendency both for women and their doctors to assign blame to whatever is seen as a defect. Obese women often believe that if they lost weight, their PMS would get better. This is not the case: PMS affects women of all sizes, shapes, and weights.

Women home with children often assume that if they had jobs outside the home, their PMS would improve, while women with careers say, "I envy women at home because they don't have to function on a job. They have it easier." The reality is that women at home with or without children have PMS; women with careers, even very successful careers, have PMS. There may be other reasons for getting or giving up jobs, but curing PMS shouldn't be one of them. PMS is not caused by housework, children, or professions.

Mental illness does not cause PMS. Women can be emotionally disturbed with or without PMS. These disturbances occur regardless of the menstrual period. Women who are emotionally healthy, aware of their feelings, and able to cope well can have severe PMS. However, PMS can be more devastating to women whose sense of identity and control are already precarious.

Perfectionism and PMS do seem to be related. Women who maintain exceptionally high standards of behavior and control appear to be more easily shaken by finding themselves periodically unable to meet those standards. PMS is probably not more common in these women, but they often have a more difficult time dealing with it.

PMS is not caused by other people. It may be worse in stressful situations and in dysfunctional relationships, but PMS resides within the individual woman who experiences the symptoms.

CHAPTER 5

❈

PMS and the Perimenopausal Transition

I could be called a late bloomer when it comes to PMS—my symptoms were very mild until I turned forty. Then I started feeling much more anxious and irritable for a full two weeks before my period. I often felt intensely angry with my husband and children, many times when they weren't doing or saying anything that unusual. Diet and exercise weren't enough. Something had changed in my body.

One day I realized that my PMS was gone. I was walking past an ice cream store and realized I hadn't craved chocolate in a while. I kind of missed that feeling. Then I remembered I hadn't been irritable either, not in the way I used to be when I was premenstrual. Come to think of it, I hadn't had a period in a couple of months. And I wasn't pregnant!

Have you noticed that as we get older, our definitions of "young," "middle-aged," and "older" seem to change? And they always change in the same direction, that is, the age creeps upward. A teenager thinks thirty is old! A thirty-five-year-old thinks thirty is young.

Our culture favors youth. We don't look forward to growing older and try to hide the telltale external signs of age. We often face the internal changes of growing older with apprehension. Our faces change; our ovaries change; our emotions change; our circumstances change. None of these changes occur in isolation.

Menopause occurs throughout the world. For some women it is a smooth and barely noticed transition; for others it is catastrophic. The end of menstruation is experienced and expressed differently in different cultures and countries. Whether these differences are a reflection of culture, environment, personality, or genes is unknown. Probably they are a combination of all of these.

"The change" has long been the code name for menopause. But technically menopause is the prolonged absence of a menstrual period, so it is really a retrospective diagnosis. You don't really know it has happened until it is past. Menopause, the ending of menstrual periods, occurs when the ovaries stop producing sufficient estrogen. It can occur naturally with growing older, or it can occur suddenly, as with surgical removal of the ovaries. Women on hormone replacement may not even know when menopause occurs because the hormones themselves can stop or prolong menstrual periods.

Women with PMS often want to know what will happen with menopause, and when. PMS is defined by its relationship to the menstrual cycle. The approach of menopause can make PMS better or worse. We don't yet know why, or how to predict what will happen or when. For some women, it just goes away.

Much of what we have come to think of as menopause is really *perimenopause*—that time of menstrual-pattern changes leading *up to* and *around* the cessation of menstruation. Periods change; they become heavier or lighter; they occur more frequently or less frequently; they may be more painful or less painful. Changes in ovarian function are reflected by those of menstruation, sometimes for several years before periods end. In recent years we have come to understand much more about those years preceding menopause and to see that some of the symptoms you experience are really those of PMS.

Some changes in women's reproductive function occur suddenly, as with the *event* of the first period (menarche), or with ovulation each month. Others, however, are gradual ones. Perimenopause is not a single event; there is no marker. It's another term for "moving toward menopause." Menopause *is* an event, however, in the case of surgical removal of the ovaries.

Understanding where you are in relation to menopause is even more confusing today than in the past. The hormones used in replacement therapies often affect bleeding. They may interfere with ovulation and menstruation so you won't get a period, or they may cause you to have a period. If you don't have troubling symptoms, then it may not matter much whether or not you are having periods, other than for practical considerations. Some women are sensitive to the medications used for hormone replacement and may actually develop PMS-like symptoms from taking them.

What Happens in Perimenopause

The average age for menopause is between forty-nine and fifty-four, although some women reach menopause in their early forties or late fifties. Perimenopause can begin as early as age thirty-five, but for most women the perimenopausal transition occurs when they are in their late forties.

Perimenopause is a time of gradual changes as your body winds down its reproductive function. The ovaries begin producing less progesterone and estrogen, responding only erratically to pituitary signals. The decline in progesterone and estrogen levels is accompanied by a rise in follicle-stimulating hormone (FSH) and luteinizing hormone (LH). This increase is the body's attempt to stimulate eggs, just as it has done with each menstrual cycle.

As your body slows its production of key reproductive hormones, ovulation may become erratic. It may occur irregularly—at times of the month when you are not expecting it, not at all some months, or more than once during other months.

Along with the shifts in progesterone, estrogen, FSH, and LH, your body's supply of testosterone also declines during perimenopause, although only slightly. Testosterone is a hormone produced by both men and women, although women produce much less. Testosterone is usually thought of as the male sex hormone, although it continues to be produced by women in small amounts throughout their lives.

Perimenopause Symptoms

Perimenopausal symptoms may include:

- Lighter, shorter periods, or spotting
- Heavy periods with clotting
- Irregular menstrual cycle; skipped periods
- Insomnia
- Fatigue
- Weight gain
- Mood swings; increased anxiety or depression
- Lack of libido
- Dry skin and hair
- Vaginal dryness
- Stress incontinence—urine loss upon coughing, laughing, or sneezing

Hormone Balance in Perimenopause

Women approaching menopause today are far more educated about their bodies than the generations that preceded them. They are also a group who have demanded that the medical community take seriously their experiences and perceptions. They are well-read about estrogen and want to understand and make appropriate decisions regarding replacement therapy. While most of the medical focus has been on estrogen decline at menopause, there are other hormonal changes occurring at the same time. During perimenopause, progesterone may decline first, long before estrogen tapers off. Many symptoms of perimenopause, notably anxiety, irritability, and menstrual-cycle irregularity, are associated with either how much progesterone is in the body or how the body uses progesterone.

Predictability and Control

Some of you may sail through menopause easily, barely noticing changes in your body, while others will become aware of increasing symptoms they had come to recognize as PMS. Some women may not realize their perimenopausal transition has begun until they remark that their PMS symptoms either become markedly worse or appear for the first time. For other women, a large measure of their ability to recognize and manage PMS symptoms is suddenly gone during perimenopause, because their cycles become sporadic and less predictable.

Some women have shorter menstrual cycles during perimenopause, with a period every twenty-three or twenty-four days. More frequent periods can mean that PMS symptoms occur more often, an unsettling change. It's also not uncommon to skip periods during perimenopause. Delayed or skipped periods can create a time of uncertainty about pregnancy, probably prompting the purchase of a lot of home pregnancy tests.

For some women, symptoms of depression, which have always been a part of their PMS, become more severe and more extended.

> *It seems like I have fewer good days every month now. I used to count on feeling very energetic and optimistic the week after my period, like I could take on the world. I don't have those bursts of energy often anymore, and I sometimes feel like my symptoms have no sooner ended than they're back again.*

Special Considerations for Perimenopausal Women

Women in the perimenopausal time frame can definitely have PMS. It's not a one-or-the-other situation. However, women in perimenopause may not have symptoms that follow a perfectly cyclical pattern. Self-help may require extra patience and flexibility as their hormonal profile continues to change.

For example, perimenopausal women often respond very well physically to a diet, exercise, and stress-reduction program, reporting that breast tenderness, bloating, and fatigue are improved. However, emotional symptoms such as anxiety and irritability can be more stubborn to manage during perimenopause. It's important not to judge yourself or to assume you aren't doing something right. You may need to consider complementing your self-help program with other treatments.

Remember, the question of PMS and menopause, like the larger questions of mind and body and of biology and environment, is not an either/or. We live in biological environments, internal and external ones.

We have our chemistry, our families, our work, and our spiritual lives. Our minds, our personalities, our decisions and values all occur in a biological and social matrix. Perimenopause is about hormones; it is about getting older; it is about being a woman experiencing change. As with all other aspects of our lives, our environments, both biological and cultural, affect us, but they do not entirely determine our feelings and actions.

❀

CHAPTER 6

Premenstrual Magnification (PMM)

My asthma is usually set off by colds, so I am always susceptible to attacks. I have realized that the ones that send me to the emergency room seem to occur the day before my period starts. Sometimes I even begin to menstruate while I am still in the ER.

Two years ago I was diagnosed as having lupus. Premenstrually it usually gives me more problems, especially with my skin rashes. My joints ache more, too.

Premenstrual magnification (PMM) is the increased severity premenstrually of a condition that may be present throughout the menstrual cycle.

The premenstrual magnification of other illnesses and the occurrence of some illnesses predominantly in the premenstrual phase are not new phenomena. Aside from all the ancient myths, modern medicine in the 1930s and 40s reported scarlet fever and diphtheria as being variable in relation to the menstrual cycle. But a renewed interest in women's health makes PMM yet another new frontier in understanding the menstrual cycle and its effects on women.

It is important to understand the relationship between PMS and PMM.

· Both are related to the menstrual cycle.
· In PMS, symptoms occur *only* premenstrually and disappear with the onset of menstruation.
· In PMM, symptoms *worsen* premenstrually but improve gradually with the onset of menstruation.
· Both can be present at the same time.
· Both are real.
· PMS goes away quickly with the onset of menstruation. PMM symptoms linger and improve slowly over a few days. They rarely go away totally.

The last fifteen years have seen greater interest and understanding about PMS. However, PMM has largely been ignored. One reason for this is that studying the menstrual cycle turns out to be quite difficult, because it is changing all the time. Research is most easily done in a situation in which it is possible to keep almost all conditions of the study the same and then alter a minimum number of factors. In that way, differences in results can be explained by differences in treatments.

As described earlier, women were often excluded from studies of drugs, precisely because the menstrual cycle made the studies more difficult, "confusing" the results. Many practitioners had found that their female patients sometimes responded differently to drugs than male patients. This was especially true for dosages of antidepressants. Menstrual-cycle variations in drug responses have also been seen with antiseizure and antiasthmatic medications. New federal guidelines now require that women be included in drug studies, so the problem of drug regimens should lessen with time.

Women with premenstrual magnification of their symptoms face some of the same problems as women with PMS twenty years ago. They may not be believed; they may be told that they do not really have a cyclic disturbance related to their menstrual periods. They are turned away from help for PMS because they don't have a symptom-free week each month. Thus they often do not receive the help they need for the condition they have.

Women who have premenstrual magnification of an illness or who tend to get sick with their periods frequently also have some characteristics of PMS. There seems to be a relationship between premenstrual distress and vulnerability to infections.

A Look at the Evidence

· Asthma attacks may occur more frequently in the days before the onset of menstruation. Pulmonary-function tests of asthmatic women have shown a menstrual-cycle variability. In some women, asthma attacks are more severe premenstrually.

· Seizures may occur more frequently and more severely premenstrually. The blood levels of several of the common antiseizure medications can vary as a result of the menstrual cycle. This fluctuation may be responsible for differences in seizure activity over the course of the menstrual cycle.

· Migraine headaches are more frequent and more severe around menstruation. They usually occur just before or in the first two or three days of menstruation.

· Skin disorders may worsen premenstrually. Allergic conditions change, and skin may be more sensitive and sometimes may even change color from contact with some metals in jewelry. Acne is well known to flare up in relation to hormone fluctuation.

· Infections can occur more frequently or worsen in relation to the phase of the menstrual cycle. These include:

  · vaginal yeast infections
  · bladder infections
  · toxic shock syndrome
  · abscesses
  · skin infections
  · herpes

Women with PMM, unlike those with PMS, may be ill throughout the entire month, but they are worse premenstrually. Whether they suffer from asthma, epilepsy, diabetes, depression, arthritis, or almost any other disease, their difficulties increase premenstrually and are then partially relieved with the onset of menstruation. Unlike women with PMS, when these women get their periods, they do not have the dramatic relief from all their symptoms because the underlying disorder is still there.

The chart on page 79 illustrates this pattern of symptoms.

In a good month I'm usually very tired ten days before I start bleeding. I wake up tired and go to bed tired. In a bad

*month I'm tired almost every day. I will sleep an hour at
lunch and then anywhere from one to two hours when I get
home from work. I've been mildly depressed as long as I can
remember.*

Treatment of PMM is not always the same as for PMS. The underlying
disorder must usually be treated first, independent of PMS. Treating
PMM depression tends only to remove the underlying depression but still
leaves a sometimes severe premenstrual fluctuation of mood. So along
with treatment for the constant depression, treatment for the PMS then
becomes necessary. Likewise, with asthma or seizures, the underlying condition must be addressed independent of PMS.

Women with PMM often describe *feeling different* premenstrually, even
though their symptoms are present all month.

*I know I'm depressed other times, but it feels different pre-
menstrually. It takes on a characteristic of doom, impending
doom.*

Although it might seem to an observer or health care practitioner that
a woman is ill all the time, she may feel her illness more acutely premenstrually.

Women with PMM need to know they are not isolated cases of a rare
disorder but rather that they share a common experience. The lesson of
PMM is to pay attention to women about what they are *feeling.* Then,
when their symptoms don't seem to make sense or fit into previous beliefs
about a disease, the challenge is to question the beliefs, not the women.

CHAPTER 7

❀

PMS
and Mental Illness

I was examining a patient who had come to see me for PMS, and I mentioned to her that the American Psychiatric Association was establishing a diagnosis for PMS. Her first reaction was, "Thank God someone is looking at it." Then she reflected for a moment and said, "Oh, no! They're saying I'm crazy."

Because some of the symptoms of PMS are emotional, and because the menstrual cycle may affect psychiatric disorders, there is often confusion in sorting out the differences between PMS and mental illness. Intensification of psychiatric illness, especially depression, is common. But as described earlier, it is a premenstrual magnification of an underlying disorder, not PMS. Much of the research about PMS has been conducted on women with depression and is therefore not reflective of the general population of women with PMS.

Some of the confusion results from the history of PMS research in the United States. Many of the earliest researchers to take an interest in PMS were psychiatrists who were trained and experienced in depression research. Therefore, depression was what they first examined. Because of the research criteria and process of selection, the women studied tended to be more impaired and more vulnerable to depression and other psychiatric illness.

PMS as a diagnosis was new at the time, and few researchers or doctors had much clinical experience with the problem. Following up on the reports in the media of women whose extreme violence was attributed to hormones, the researchers set about finding that population to study. They looked for women who were fine for two weeks of the month, then violent, suicidal, or otherwise seriously impaired for the last two weeks of their cycles. They were looking for a stereotype that didn't exist. The women they eventually studied suffered more from mental illness than from PMS.

Research has also been flawed because the processes used to identify subjects often led to women with PMS being excluded, instead of included. A prolonged process of assessment, while intended to increase the accuracy of the research, has resulted in some major weaknesses, especially with regard to PMS and mental illness.

1. Many women with PMS are not good at filling out a form every day for two to three months without receiving any treatment or support. When women with PMS are premenstrual, they are often disorganized, moody, and irritable—and not highly motivated to complete forms. When they are not premenstrual, they do not really believe the problem will come back again.

2. Information about PMS and help for it are much more available today than they were in the early 1980s. Most women with PMS are able to get relief either through self-help methods or from their health care providers. Therefore, those who enter studies often have more severe PMS that has not responded to treatment, and therefore represent a somewhat different group of women.

3. Research has often been conducted at psychiatric facilities. Therefore, those women who entered the studies often saw themselves in terms of psychiatric illness or were at least more familiar with psychiatric care.

The result is a blurring of distinction between PMS and psychiatric illness, as much of the PMS research is conducted on women with more past or concurrent psychiatric illness than is seen in the general population of women with PMS.

Premenstrual Dysphoric Disorder

In the 1980s the American Psychiatric Association in conjunction with the American Psychological Association began to develop research criteria to use in studying PMS. Their first attempt was a diagnosis published in 1987, *late luteal phase dysphoric disorder (LLPDD)*. In 1994 they changed that diagnosis to *premenstrual dysphoric disorder (PDD)*. However, the researchers and clinicians who developed these diagnoses are clear in distinguishing these disorders from PMS. The differences lie in severity, the presence of other disorders at the same time, and spread of symptoms beyond the premenstrual phase.

Confusion persists, partly because of the overlapping of symptoms; of stigma associated with mental illness, which may influence people away from psychiatric diagnoses; and of insurance rules, which may favor or discriminate against psychiatric illnesses.

PMM further confuses the distinction. Many women with chronic depression are more depressed premenstrually. This is premenstrual magnification (PMM) of an underlying disorder (in this case, depression). For some women, the menstrual cycle acts as a destabilizing factor, exacerbating an underlying state or condition. If you are depressed, you may become more depressed. If you are violent, you may become more violent.

Psychiatric Disorders Affected by the Menstrual Cycle

Psychiatric conditions can be affected by the menstrual cycle. The following disorders can be magnified premenstrually.

DEPRESSION: Women with depression may be worse premenstrually. Fleeting suicidal thoughts can become plans to take one's life.

ANOREXIA AND BULIMIA: The premenstrual phase impacts negatively on many women's body image and self-esteem. Women can find themselves looking in the mirror, suddenly unhappy with their skin, hair, or shape. For women who have a disorder that is linked with negative body images, the premenstrual phase compounds their dissatisfaction with their bodies. Then add the cravings for sweets that accompany the premenstrual state, and it is clear why women with eating disorders may be much worse premenstrually. Bulimics binge and purge more. Anorexics struggle more to maintain control at this time of month.

AGORAPHOBIA: Agoraphobia is the irrational fear of leaving familiar places, or home. The origin of the term is from the Greek, *agora*—"marketplace," and *phobia*—"fear." Historically, it was a fear of the marketplace. Agoraphobics are indeed afraid of leaving home. Many, however, are able to leave, albeit with effort, during part of the month but premenstrually are homebound.

OBSESSIVE-COMPULSIVE DISORDER: For some women OCD, a combination of obsessive thoughts and/or compulsive behaviors, becomes worse premenstrually.

PSYCHOSIS: Psychosis is a broad term encompassing various serious mental illnesses. Some of the more flagrant symptoms, like hearing voices, may be intensified during the premenstrual phase, especially just prior to the onset of menstruation.

ALCOHOLISM AND DRUG DEPENDENCE: Substance abuse may also be more of a problem premenstrually. Alcohol affects women differently over the course of the menstrual cycle, as described earlier. In addition, there is the problem of decreased sense of control, greater impulsivity, more cravings, and more temptation to self-medicate for the symptoms and escape from the negative feelings about oneself.

There are other psychiatric illnesses that may be affected by the menstrual cycle. There is not always a clear-cut distinction as to what is PMS and what is mental illness, especially since symptoms overlap. Anyone experiencing serious symptoms should seek help; no one should allow biases about mental illness to keep her from seeking help. The purpose of distinguishing between PMS, PMM, and psychiatric illness is to better direct treatment. It is not to judge or to divide illnesses into good ones or bad, self-induced or caused by factors beyond one's control.

CHAPTER 8

❀

Diagnosis

Do You Have PMS?

There is no mystery to the diagnosis of PMS. In fact, it is most easily made on the basis of the "Aha!" experience. If you read stories about women with PMS and say to yourself, "That's me," then you probably have PMS. If the same stories and descriptions don't ring any bells in you then you probably don't.

Currently there are no reliable chemical, physical, or psychological tests to determine PMS. There is charting, which a woman does herself, and there are several diagnostic criteria that are suggestive of PMS but not definitive. Even charting can be difficult to evaluate because there are women who may have some symptoms all month long but who still insist that they "feel different" premenstrually. PMS is an experience that a woman either has or doesn't have. The only absolute criteria is the presence of the symptoms in the premenstrual phase of her cycle and their dramatic alleviation with the onset of her menses.

Common Characteristics of PMS

While the many symptoms of PMS include some that are common and some that are rare, usually one or more of the following collection of characteristics describe women with PMS.

1. Onset following puberty, pregnancy, extreme weight loss with temporary cessation of periods, use of birth control pills, tubal ligation, ovarian surgery, or hysterectomy.

2. Worsening with pregnancy (it can be increasingly severe with subsequent pregnancies), cessation of periods from weight loss, use of birth control pills, tubal ligation, ovarian surgery, hysterectomy.

3. Miscarriage and toxemia of pregnancy seem to be more common among women with PMS.

4. Postpartum depression may be followed quickly by PMS and occurs more frequently among women who have had PMS prior to their pregnancies.

5. Pregnancy is usually a positive experience for women with PMS, especially after the first trimester. Often they describe being pregnant as the one time they feel wonderful. This characteristic is ironic because women have at times become pregnant as a solution to depression only to discover that their PMS is worse after they give birth.

6. Menstruation is more often painless, dysmenorrhea unusual. There is no particular cycle length or type of menstrual bleeding characteristic of PMS. Cycles may be long or short, regular or irregular; bleeding may be light or heavy, with or without clots.

7. Women with PMS who take birth control pills often experience headache, weight gain, and depression as side effects and may have to discontinue the pills. Other women find that contraceptives relieve their PMS.

8. Acute symptoms (migraine headaches, panic attacks, epilepsy, depression, et cetera) often follow long gaps between meals—that is, five hours in the day or thirteen hours overnight.

9. Food cravings and binges can be quite severe for women with PMS. Women with mild difficulties may say, "I always know when my period is due because I find myself eyeing chocolate and touching potato-chip bags in the grocery store." Eating disorders are most difficult to control at this time because self-control is at its lowest. For women who are dieting, this is a most difficult time because they tend to binge and then hate them-

selves for failing at their diet; then they try to fast, which may bring on hypoglycemic symptoms.

10. Women can be much more sensitive to alcohol premenstrually. In addition, some women turn to alcohol for relief from tension. Combined with their increased sensitivity and with alcohol's depressive effect, this may lead to more drinking and depression. Furthermore, certain women who have repeatedly turned to alcohol for relief of PMS symptoms have become alcoholics.

11. Sex-drive changes premenstrually can take the form of either an increase or decrease in sexual desire. Some women lose any desire for sex premenstrually while others have an increase, especially in the few days just before their periods (see Chapter 19).

12. Women with PMS typically experience a sense of relief when they get their periods. This relief usually comes on abruptly, sometime between twelve hours prior to bleeding and twenty-four hours after the period begins. Even when the menses itself is painful or exhausting, women usually say they feel much better as soon as they bleed. They say that "the cloud has been lifted."

Charting PMS Symptoms

Charting symptoms is an important key to diagnosis, since it provides a picture of when the symptoms are occurring in relation to the menses, which symptoms are related to the cycle, and which are present at other times too.

It is wise to approach charting with a sense of curiosity and exploration rather than a desire to prove or disprove whether you have PMS. Invariably, women find that some of what they thought was PMS also occurs at other times and that other symptoms thought to be irrelevant actually occur premenstrually. Charting should not be oppressive, but for women who want to know precisely when and which symptoms may be related to PMS, keeping track is one of the best ways to get that information. And remember that charting is just a record of *your experience.*

STEP-BY-STEP CHARTING: Charting itself can be simple or complicated, depending on what is being recorded and how much energy you have to devote to the task. The simplest form is like Chart 1, which follows. As a practical matter, the chart has eight columns instead of twelve to give you more room to mark symptoms. A wall calendar or small yearly calendar can also be useful. What is important is to be able to see graphically when symptoms are occurring in relation to your menstrual cycle.

In Chart 1 the numbers along the left margin represent the days of the month. Mark the individual months across the top. Note the dates of your menstrual period with an *M*. If you have spotting for a day or two before or after your period, mark those days with an *S*.

CHART 1

SYMPTOMS   INITIALS

1. ———————————————————————— ————————

2. ———————————————————————— ————————   Menstruation: Ⓜ

3. ———————————————————————— ————————   Date charting began: ——————————————

MONTHS

1							
2							
3							
4							
5							
6							
7							
8							
9							
10							
11							
12							
13							
14							
15							
16							
17							
18							
19							
20							
21							
22							
23							
24							
25							
26							
27							
28							
29							
30							
31							

CHART 2

If your period was from January 15 through 20, February 14 through 18, and March 17 through 21, your chart will look like Chart 2. Although the average length of the menstrual cycle is twenty-eight days, it varies considerably from woman to woman, and the length may also change at different times in a woman's life. Cycle length is not related to PMS, nor is the regularity of the cycle, nor the number of days of bleeding. Traditionally, the cycle is numbered beginning with the first day of bleeding of one period and ending with the first day of bleeding of the next period.

Note that here the cycle beginning January 15 was thirty days, the next one thirty-one days.

CHART 2

SYMPTOMS   INITIALS

1. _____ _____

2. _____ _____   Menstruation: (M)

3. _____ _____   Date charting began: _____

MONTHS

	January		February		March										
1				(18)		(16)									
2				(19)		(17)									
3				(20)		(18)									
4				(21)		(19)									
5				(22)		(20)									
6				(23)		(21)									
7				(24)		(22)									
8				(25)		(23)									
9				(26)		(24)									
10				(27)		(25)									
11				(28)		(26)									
12				(29)		(27)									
13				(30)		(28)									
14			(M)	(1)		(29)									
15	(M)	(1)	(M)	(2)		(30)									
16	(M)	(2)	(M)	(3)		(31)									
17	(M)	(3)	(M)	(4)	(M)	(1)									
18	(M)	(4)	(M)	(5)	(M)	(2)									
19	(M)	(5)		(6)	(M)	(3)									
20	(M)	(6)		(7)	(M)	(4)									
21		(7)		(8)	(M)	(5)									
22		(8)		(9)		(6)									
23		(9)		(10)		(7)									
24		(10)		(11)		(8)									
25		(11)		(12)		(9)									
26		(12)		(13)		(10)									
27		(13)		(14)		(11)									
28		(14)		(15)		(12)									
29		(15)	✕			(13)									
30		(16)				(14)									
31		(17)				(15)									

CHART 3

If you also had breast tenderness, which you represent with a B, from January 4 through 15, February 10 through 14, and March 5 through 15, your chart would look like Chart 3.

CHART 3

SYMPTOMS   INITIALS

1. _Breast Tenderness_ _____   _B_

2. _____ _____   Menstruation: (M)

3. _____ _____   Date charting began: _____

MONTHS

	January	February	March					
1								
2								
3								
4	B							
5	B		B					
6	B		B					
7	B		B					
8	B		B					
9	B		B					
10	B	B	B					
11	B	B	B					
12	B	B	B					
13	B	B	B					
14	B	(M) B	B					
15	(M) B	(M)(M)	B					
16	(M)(M)	(M)(M)	(M)					
17	(M)(M)	(M)(M)	(M)(M)					
18	(M)(M)	(M)	(M)(M)					
19	(M)(M)		(M)(M)					
20	(M)							
21								
22								
23								
24								
25								
26								
27								
28								
29								
30		✕						
31								

CHART 4

Chart 4 shows clearly that this woman's symptoms are occurring each month prior to the onset of her period and that her tension is relieved when the period begins. It also indicates that May was an easier month, with only three days of tension. It is common for premenstrual symptoms to vary as to length, intensity, and type.

CHART 4

SYMPTOMS   INITIALS

1. *Tension* _____ __T__

2. _____ _____

3. _____ _____

Menstruation: (M)

Date charting began: _____

MONTHS

	January	February	March	April	May	June		
1								
2								
3						T		
4						T		
5			T			T		
6			T			T		
7		T	T			T		
8		T	T			T		
9	T	T	T			T		
10	T	T		T		T		
11	T	T	T	T	T	(M)		
12	T	T	T	T	T	(M)		
13	T	T	T	T	T	(M)		
14	T	T	T	T	(m)	(M)		
15	T	T	T	T	(M)			
16	T	T	(M)		(M)			
17	T	(M)	(M)	T	(M)			
18	(M)	(M)	(M)	T				
19	(M)	(M)	(M)					
20	(M)	(M)		T				
21	(M)			T				
22	(M)			T				
23				(M)				
24				(M)				
25				(M)				
26				(M)				
27				(M)				
28								
29								
30		✕						
31			✕		✕			

CHART 5

Three symptoms appear in Chart 5: breast tenderness, lethargy, and depression. Notice that the breast changes often precede the emotional ones, although this is not always true. The lethargy tends to begin about a week before and to last through one or two days of the period. The depression lifts with the onset of menstruation. Note also that in one month there were no breast symptoms at all.

CHART 5

SYMPTOMS	INITIALS
1. Breast Tenderness	B
2. Lethargy	L
3. Depression	D

Menstruation: (M)

Date charting began: _____

MONTHS

	January	February	March	April	May	June	July	August
1		B		B		B L D		
2	B	B		B	D	B L D		
3	B	B D	B D	B D	L D	B L D		
4	B	B D	B D	B D	L D	B L D		
5	B D	B L D	B D	B L D	L D	B L D		
6	B D	B L D	B D	B L D	L D	B L D		
7	B D	B L D	B L D	B L D	(M) L D	(M) L		
8	B D	B L D	B L D	B L D	(M) L	(M)		
9	B L D	B L D	B L D	B L D	(M)	(M)		
10	B L D	B L D	B L D	B L D	(M)	(M)		
11	B L D	B L D	B L D	B L D	(M)	(M)		
12	B L D	(M) L	B L D	B L D		(M)		
13	B L D	(M)	(M) L	(M) L				
14	B L D	(M)	(M)	(M)				
15	B L D	(M)	(M)	(M)				
16	(M) L		(M)	(M)				
17	(M) L		(M)					
18	(M)		(M)					
19	(M)		(M)					
20								
21								
22								
23								
24								
25								
26								
27					B			
28					B			
29		X			B			
30		X	B		B L D			
31	B	X	B	X	B L D	X		

CHART 6

On Chart 6, the woman's bloating clearly occurs only premenstrually, but you will notice that her anger has occurred at other times. There are two possible explanations. One is that further charting will show that the anger is predominantly premenstrual; the other that there are other reasons she is experiencing and expressing anger. Where there is anger at other times of the month, women often say that the premenstrual anger and depression "feels different."

CHART 6

SYMPTOMS   INITIALS
1. _Anger_ _____   _A_
2. _Depression_ _____   _D_   Menstruation: (M)
3. _Bloating_ _____   _B_   Date charting began: _____

MONTHS

	January	February	March	April	May	June	July	August
1	(M)	(M)	(M)	(M)	B D	(M)	(m)	
2	(M)	(M)	(M)	(M)	(M)	(M)	(M)	
3	(M)	(M)	(M)	(M)	(M)	(M)	(M)	
4	(M)		(M)	(M) A	(M)	(M)		
5				A	(M)			
6						A		
7						A		
8								
9								
10		A						
11		A						
12		A						
13								
14								
15								
16						A		
17				B		D A		
18				B		B D A		
19				B		B D		
20	D	B D		B		B D		
21	B D	B D				B D		
22	B D	B D		B D	A	B D		
23	B D	B D		B D	A	B		
24	B D	B D A	B	B D A	B	A B D		
25	B D A	B D A	B	B D A	B	A B D		
26	B D A	B A	B D A	B D A	B D	B		
27	B D A	B A	B D A	B D A	B D	B D		
28	B D A	B A	B D A	B D	B D	(M)		
29	B D A	✕	B D A	B D	B D	(M)		
30	(M)	✕	B D A	B D	B D	(M)		
31	(M)	✕	(M)	✕	B D	✕		

CHART 7

Another way of charting symptoms is by severity. When it isn't clear that a symptom occurs *only* premenstrually, you can chart its intensity on a scale. Instead of recording three different symptoms, a woman who is usually anxious rates the *level* of anxiety on a scale in which 1 = mild, 2 = moderate, and 3 = severe. In this way she is able to chart the relationship between the severity of her symptoms and her menstrual cycle. Although she has anxiety much of the month, it is more severe premenstrually. This is an example of PMM, premenstrual magnification.

CHART 7

SYMPTOMS	INITIALS
1. Mild	1
2. Moderate	2
3. Severe	3

Menstruation: (M)
Date charting began: _____

Anxiety

MONTHS

	January	February	March	April	May	June	July	August
1			(M)	(M) 1	(M) 3	(M) 1		
2			(M)	(M) 1	(M) 1	(M)		
3		1	(M) 1	3	(M) 1	(M)		
4		1	(M) 1	1	(M) 1	(M)		
5		1	(M) 1	1	(M)			
6		2	1	1				
7		2	2	1	1			
8		1	2	2	1			
9		1	1					
10			1					
11			1					
12		1		1				
13		1		2				
14		1	3	1				
15		2	3	1				
16			1					
17			1	3				
18	3	1	1	3				
19	3	1	3	3				
20	3	3	3	3				
21	3	3	3	2				
22	3	3	2	2				
23	3	3	3	1				
24	2	3	3	2				
25	3	1	3	3	3			
26	2	3	2	3	3			
27	3	1	2	3	3			
28	(M)	(M)	3	3	3			
29	(M)		(M) 3	3	3			
30	(M) 1		(M) 3	3	3			
31	(M) 1		(M) 1		(M)			

CHART 8

Sometimes there are so many symptoms and so little clarity as to which ones are related to the cycle that the charting must be expanded. One way is to use each chart for a separate month. Insert the symptoms across the top of the chart, and in the columns either use check marks to indicate the presence of a symptom or a scale of 1 to 3 to describe the severity of symptoms. Charts 8, 9, and 10 represent three months of charting multiple symptoms.

In January it is clear that this woman's anxiety is premenstrual. Her insomnia began premenstrually but *continued,* so only further charting will show if there is a pattern. The rage occurred three times, twice premenstrually, so this requires more charting. Headaches seemed to be scattered throughout the month. She also had what she described as "weird feelings" that she thought were only premenstrual. They consisted of slight dizziness, disorientation, and difficulty focusing. Colors seemed sharper, and her body felt slightly "strange." In January these feelings indeed occurred only premenstrually. Sinus difficulties, which she had thought to be related to her period, on charting seemed to come *after* her period began and to last into the first week postmenstrually. In January she also had a few days of nausea and marked this on the chart under "Other."

CHART 8

SYMPTOMS   INITIALS

1. _____ _____

2. _____ _____   Menstruation: (M)

3. _____ _____   Date charting began: _____

MONTHS SYMPTOMS   JANUARY   Other:

	Menstruation	Anxiety	Insomnia	Rage	Headaches	Weird feelings	Sinus	
1				✓	✓			
2					✓			
3					✓			
4					✓			
5					✓			
6								
7								
8								
9								
10								
11		✓						nausea
12		✓						
13		✓		✓				
14		✓		✓		✓		
15		✓	✓			✓		
16		✓	✓			✓		
17	(M)		✓			✓		
18	(M)		✓					
19	(M)		✓				✓	
20	(M)		✓				✓	
21	(M)		✓		✓		✓	
22			✓		✓		✓	
23			✓		✓		✓	
24					✓		✓	
25					✓			
26					✓			
27								
28					✓			
29					✓			
30								
31								

CHART 9

The February chart shows a similar pattern, with the woman's anxiety, rage, and "weird feelings" clearly premenstrual. The insomnia does not seem to be related to this woman's cycle, and sinus problems again follow the menses.

CHART 9

SYMPTOMS INITIALS

1. _____ _____

2. _____ _____ Menstruation: (M)

3. _____ _____ Date charting began: _____

~~MONTHS~~ SYMPTOMS   FEBRUARY   Other:

	Menstruation	Anxiety	Insomnia	Rage	Headaches	weird feelings	Sinus	
1								
2								
3			✓		✓			
4			✓		✓			
5								
6								
7								
8								
9								
10		✓			✓	✓		
11		✓			✓	✓		nausea
12		✓				✓		
13		✓		✓		✓		
14		✓		✓		✓		
15	(M)			✓		✓		
16	(M)			✓		✓		
17	(M)				✓			
18	(M)				✓		✓	
19					✓		✓	
20					✓		✓	
21					✓		✓	
22			✓		✓		✓	
23			✓		✓			
24			✓					
25			✓					
26			✓					
27								
28								
29								
30								
31								

CHART 10

By the third month (Chart 10) the pattern is even clearer. If you look back over the previous cycles, it is clear that the anxiety, rage, and "weird feelings" are premenstrual. Insomnia and headaches seem to occur at any time in the cycle. The nausea was premenstrual for two months but then did not recur, so it is unclear whether it is cycle-related. One episode of bingeing occurred premenstrually in March, and although this is probably cycle-related, that cannot really be determined without more charting.

CHART 10

SYMPTOMS   INITIALS

1. _____ _____

2. _____ _____   Menstruation: Ⓜ

3. _____ _____   Date charting began: _____

~~MONTHS~~ SYMPTOMS   MARCH   Other:

	Menstruation	Anxiety	Insomnia	Rage	Headaches	Weird Feelings	Sinus	
1								
2		✓			✓			
3					✓			
4					✓			
5		✓						
6								
7								
8		✓						
9								
10								
11					✓			
12					✓			
13		✓			✓	✓		
14		✓	✓	✓		✓		Bingeing
15		✓	✓	✓		✓		
16	Ⓜ	✓	✓	✓				
17	Ⓜ							
18	Ⓜ		✓					
19	Ⓜ		✓					
20			✓				✓	
21			✓				✓	
22			✓				✓	
23			✓				✓	
24			✓				✓	
25			✓				✓	
26								
27								
28								
29								
30								
31								

CHART II

Sometimes the symptoms shift in severity during the premenstrual phase. They usually begin at the time of ovulation. They may then get better for a few days before becoming severe again, or they may remain constant. In Chart II, the irritability around the twenty-second and twenty-third of each month represents a symptom related to the time of ovulation.

CHART II

SYMPTOMS   INITIALS

1. Irritability   I
2. Bloating   B
3. Depression   D

Menstruation: (M)

Date charting began: _____

MONTHS

	January	February	March	April					
1		I		D					
2		I		D					
3				D I					
4				D I					
5				D					
6			I D						
7	(M)		I D	(M)					
8	(M)		(M)	(M)					
9	(M)		(M)	(M)					
10	(M)	(M)	(M)	(M)					
11		(M)	(M)						
12		(M)	(M)						
13		(M)							
14									
15									
16									
17									
18									
19									
20									
21			I						
22	I		I D						
23	I D	I							
24	I	I							
25		I							
26		I							
27									
28	I								
29	I	✕							
30	I	✕	D	✕					
31		✕	D	✕					

CHART 12

Another way to chart symptoms is simply to use *S* to represent the presence of symptoms. In Chart 12 the pattern is one of premenstrual difficulties every other month. Symptoms can occur regularly every other month, every third or fourth month, or irregularly. Some women have a cycle in which premenstrual symptoms become increasingly severe month by month for four or five months. Then an easy month occurs, followed by increasingly severe symptoms again.

CHART 12

SYMPTOMS   INITIALS

1. Symptoms   S

2. _____ _____

3. _____ _____

Menstruation: (M)

Date charting began: _____

MONTHS

	June	July	August	September	October	November	December	January
1								
2					S			
3								
4							S	
5							S	
6					S		S	
7			S		S		S	
8			S		S		S	
9	S		S		S		S	
10	S		S				S	
11	S		S				S	
12	S		S		S	(M)		
13	S		S	(M)	S	(M)	(M)	
14	S		S	(M)	(M)	(M)	(M)	
15	S		(M)	(M)	(M)	(M)	(M)	
16	S		(M)	(M)	(M)		(M)	
17	S	(M)	(M)	(M)	(M)		(M)	
18	(M)	(M)	(M)		(M)			
19	(M)	(M)						
20	(M)	(M)						
21	(M)							
22								
23								
24								
25								
26								
27								
28								
29								
30								
31	✕			✕			✕	

CHART 13

Symptoms can be so severe that they spread into the "good weeks." When outbursts disrupt family and work, a woman may have little peaceful or balanced time left. What is important then is to separate the symptoms to gain an understanding of what is directly related to PMS and what is aftermath.

CHART 13

SYMPTOMS INITIALS

1. _Symptoms_ _____ _S_

2. _____ _____

3. _____ _____

Menstruation: (M)

Date charting began: _____

MONTHS

	January	February	March	April				
1		S	S	S				
2		S	S	S				
3		S	S	S				
4		S	S	S				
5		S	S	S				
6		S	S	S				
7		S	S	S				
8		S	S	S				
9		S	S	S				
10		S	S	S				
11		S	S	S				
12		S	S	S				
13		S	S	S				
14		S	S	(M) S				
15		(M) S	(M) S	(M) S				
16		(M) S	(m) S	(m) S				
17		(M) S	(M) S	(M)				
18	(M)	(m) S	(M) S					
19	(M)	(M)						
20	(M)							
21	(M)							
22	(M)		S					
23		S	S					
24		S	S					
25		S	S					
26	S	S	S					
27	S	S	S					
28	S	S	S					
29	S	✕	S					
30	S	✕	S					
31	S	✕	S	✕				

CHART 14

Postmenstrual headaches, typically beginning on Day 3 through Day 6 of the cycle, are not part of PMS. They do, however, occur in women who tend to be headache-prone and who may also have some headaches premenstrually. Although these headaches are related to the menstrual cycle, little is known about why they occur when they do.

CHART 14

SYMPTOMS   INITIALS

1. _Headache_   _H_

2. _____ _____   Menstruation: (M)

3. _____ _____   Date charting began: _____

MONTHS

	October	November	December					
1								
2								
3								
4		H						
5								
6								
7								
8								
9								
10								
11	(M)							
12	(M)	(M)						
13	(M) H	(M)	(M)					
14	(M) H	(M)	(M)					
15	H	(M) H	(M) H					
16	H	H	(M) H					
17	H	H	(M) H					
18		H	(M) H					
19			H					
20								
21								
22								
23								
24	H							
25	H							
26								
27								
28								
29								
30								
31		X						

CHART 15

This is the chart of a woman who has had a hysterectomy but whose ovaries were not removed. Although there is no *M* for menses, she has cyclic symptoms. When this analysis is combined with a temperature chart showing ovulation, the relationship between symptoms and ovulation becomes clearer.

CHART 15

SYMPTOMS   INITIALS

1. _Symptoms_____ __S__

2. _____ _____

3. _____ _____

Menstruation: ⊗

Date charting began: _____

MONTHS   Hysterectomy

	January	February	March	April	May			
1								
2			S					
3			S					
4			S		S			
5			S		S			
6			S		S			
7		S	S	S	S			
8	S	S	S	S	S			
9	S	S	S	S	S			
10	S	S		S	S			
11	S	S		S	S			
12	S	S		S	S			
13	S	S		S	S			
14	S			S	S			
15	S			S	S			
16	S			S	S			
17	S			S				
18	S			S				
19				S				
20								
21								
22								
23								
24								
25								
26								
27								
28								
29		X						
30		X						
31		X		X				

Patterns of Symptoms

The charts below show the most general patterns common to PMS in relation to the menstrual cycle. Typically, when the cycle is longer, the symptoms begin later. It is usually assumed that a woman ovulates fourteen days prior to her next menstrual period, but sometimes women ovulate at other times as well.

CHART 16

In this case the symptoms appear at ovulation, then diminish or disappear, and then recur shortly before menses, ending with the onset of bleeding.

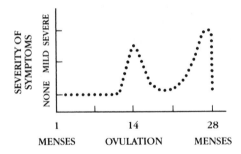

CHART 17

This chart illustrates gradually increasing premenstrual symptoms ending with menstruation.

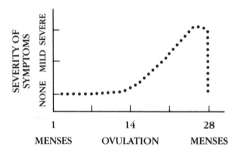

CHART 18

Here the symptoms become severe with ovulation and remain so until menses.

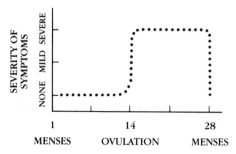

CHART 19

Some symptoms, especially headache, tend to extend into the menstrual time, through the first two or three days of the period.

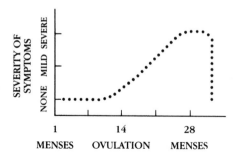

CHART 20

In cases of premenstrual magnification, symptoms are present throughout the cycle but are more severe premenstrually.

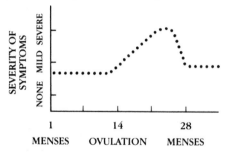

Ovulation

When it is not clear that symptoms are related to ovulation, as in long cycles, irregular cycles, or after hysterectomy when menses isn't present at all, you can chart ovulation. This is done by taking your temperature daily immediately upon awakening. A special thermometer, called a basal body thermometer, is useful for this because it measures temperature changes in tenths of a degree, which are hard to read on a regular thermometer. Basal body thermometers can be purchased at any drugstore. You must take your temperature before getting out of bed. Even mild activity can raise your temperature enough to skew the results. Sickness or stress can also skew the results, so note these on the chart.

When basal body temperature is charted, ovulation is noted by a shift in temperature over several days. A woman's basal body temperature, or "resting" temperature, is slightly lower in the first part of her cycle and then rises one half to one degree after ovulation. Some women use temperature charting to determine when to avoid or have intercourse, since ovulation is the time of greatest fertility. In charting for PMS, all you need is a general sense of when ovulation has occurred, so don't worry if you miss a day or two.

Usually PMS is related to cycles in which ovulation has occurred, but it can also occur in the absence of ovulation, as when the ovaries have been removed. The following charts show the occurrence of ovulation:

CHART 21

Ovulation is noted by the drop and then sharp rise in temperature around Day 14 or 15. Typically the temperature returns to its baseline approximately when menstruation begins.

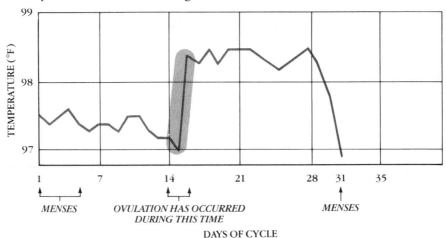

DAYS OF CYCLE

CHART 22

If the baseline average temperature remains the same throughout the cycle, ovulation has not occurred. However, you can get a period even if you have not ovulated. And you can have PMS in a cycle in which you have not ovulated.

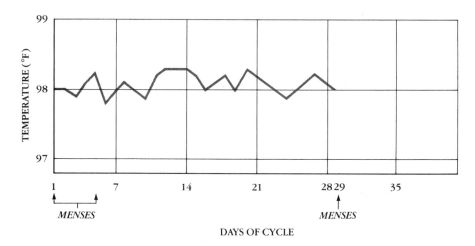

DAYS OF CYCLE

CHART 23

Ovulation usually occurs fourteen days *before* the next period, but sometimes women ovulate earlier or later than that. This chart represents a cycle in which ovulation occurred around Day 9 or 10 of the cycle. If this woman has symptoms early in the month, around Day 8 to 10, they may very well be premenstrual.

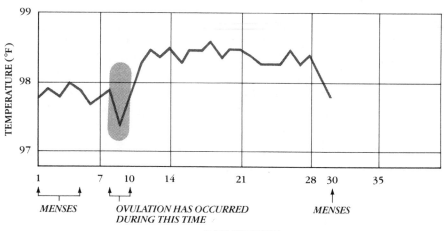

DAYS OF CYCLE

CHART 24

Here ovulation is occurring at the expected time, Day 25, for a long cycle (forty days).

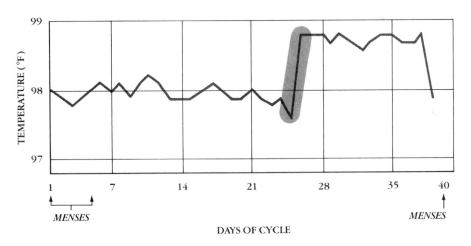

CHARTS 25 AND 26

Comparing temperature charts with symptom charts can be useful for women with irregular periods or when symptoms don't seem to make sense in terms of the cycle. The woman whose charts follow had symptoms beginning Day 6 in January and Day 16 in February. She then skipped a period in March but had symptoms on Day 42, which began at the end of February. She then had her period sixteen days after her symptoms began. In comparing the temperature charts she was keeping (Chart 26) with her symptom chart (Chart 25), it is clear that the onset of symptoms each month correlated with the days of the cycle on which she ovulated for each of those three cycles. The erratic presence of symptoms is explained by means of these charts. If, for example, ovulation had occurred around January 24 to 25, then the three days of symptoms earlier that month could not be attributed to PMS.

Remember that the temperature chart is recording days of the cycle, while the symptoms are being charted by days of the month.

CHART 25

SYMPTOMS   INITIALS

1. _Symptoms_ _____   _S_

2. _____   _____   Menstruation: (M)

3. _____   _____   Date charting began: _____

MONTHS

	January	February	March	April				
1		(M)						
2		(M)						
3		(M)						
4		(M)						
5								
6								
7				S				
8				S				
9				S				
10				S				
11				S				
12				S				
13	(M)			S				
14	(M)			S				
15	(M)			S				
16	(M)	S		S				
17		S		S				
18	S	S		S				
19	S	S		S				
20	S	S		S				
21		S		S				
22		S		(M)				
23		S		(M)				
24		S		(M)				
25		(M)		(M)				
26		(M)						
27	S	(M)						
28	S	(M)						
29	S							
30	S							
31	S							

CHART 26

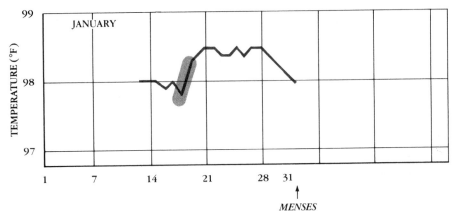

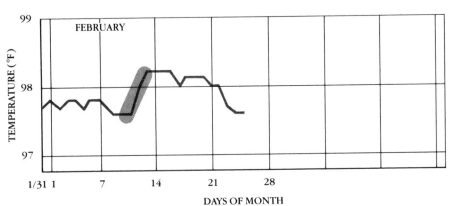

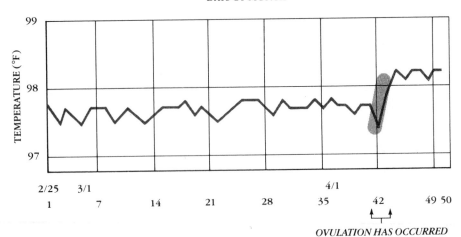

PART II

Treatment of PMS

CHAPTER 9

❀

Managing PMS

Recognizing that my symptoms were related to my menstrual cycle was a great relief. Being able to anticipate weepy or angry feelings gave me a sense of freedom—I learned about what I could do to manage these symptoms, yet I also felt safer because I knew why they were happening.

I more or less ignored my PMS symptoms for years because they were relatively mild. When they became noticeably more intense in my late thirties, I knew I had to do something. Changing the way I ate was the first thing I did, and it made a big difference right away.

How do you treat PMS?

First, you treat a *woman* who has PMS. As overwhelming as PMS may be at times, a woman is more than her dysfunctional condition. You treat the PMS within the context of her whole life, including her lifestyle, personal values, anxieties, support systems, and patience with the process.

Second, PMS symptoms are not, per se, cured—they are successfully *managed* with self-care, medication, or a combination of both, depending on the individual woman and her needs.

Here are some general principles of PMS management:

· No single method for managing PMS symptoms works for everyone. There is no silver bullet or cure, but most women with PMS find significant symptom relief when they begin a self-care program of diet, exercise, and nutritional supplements.

- PMS does not seem to like to go away. It often worsens with age (see Chapter 5), and a woman's PMS-management program may need to be refined or adjusted as symptoms persist or return or as new ones emerge.
- Success with any PMS-management program can be uneven, with results inconsistent from time to time.
- Nothing is wrong with wanting total relief from all PMS symptoms all the time, but it may not be possible.
- A woman often seeks help for PMS at a time of crisis for her and those around her. PMS can become a flash point for her situation, with all issues and problems attributed to her condition. Therefore, it's important to sort out which symptoms are related to PMS and which are unrelated but simultaneously present.
- Because of the emotional manifestations of PMS, its relief often creates unexpected changes in the woman's relationships to others. These shifts may not always be smooth. People adjust to their own illness, disability, and weakness, as do those around them. The readjustment to health and strength can be a challenge to everyone.
- Studies on PMS treatment show conflicting or inconclusive results, partly due to varying standards on selecting research subjects.
- Medical practitioners may be less informed about PMS than a woman who has taken time to educate herself about the subject. While understanding and acceptance of PMS among practitioners has grown in the last decade, you may need to take a very active role in educating your provider.
- There are several stages in coming to terms with PMS as well as in managing it. They may occur in any order: denial of PMS, relief that PMS is "real," blame, anger, and/or acceptance.
- PMS was long kept a secret because of silence concerning women's problems. Women thought themselves crazy and were unable to support one another. When that silence was broken, it was the beginning of a powerful way for women to find solutions and support for PMS by sharing their experiences with one another.
- The historical lesson of PMS is that women have not been listened to and have allowed others to define their reality. As part of your PMS-management program, it is important to keep careful records and notes

as to what *feels* better or worse. If a particular step isn't working, it isn't because you imagine it isn't working.

• Compassion for oneself is necessary in dealing with PMS.

PMS management falls into five major categories:

1. Self-care, including diet (Chapter 10), exercise (Chapter 11), and stress management (Chapter 12).

2. Nonprescription remedies such as vitamins, herbs, and nutritional supplements (Chapter 13).

3. Prescription medications, including progesterone (Chapter 14) and other prescription medications (Chapter 15).

4. Alternative therapies such as acupuncture and massage (Chapter 16).

5. Psychotherapy (Chapter 17), and support systems (Chapter 18) including both leaderless support groups and individual or group psychotherapy.

These PMS-management categories are detailed in the following chapters.

CHAPTER 10

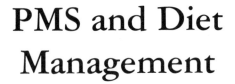

PMS and Diet Management

"Doctor, I'll do anything to get rid of these feelings."
"Then give up sugar and caffeine."
"Anything but that!"

My medical training was rather conventional. I'd been taught that people who worried about what they ate were a bit disturbed and very self-absorbed. I believed that.

But foods can and do affect our moods, and not always consistently. Caffeine stimulates adults, but may slow down children. Alcohol may pleasantly relax us, or make us agitated. It is not at all clear why foods affect PMS. PMS is a fluctuating state, and it may be that mood-affecting substances increase the fluctuations and their volatility. Eliminating some foods for a PMS diet is not a matter of virtue or of weight-loss. It is a matter of avoiding foods and substances that contribute to a roller coaster of mood changes in women with PMS.

The following dietary suggestions are based on my experience with thousands of women whose PMS has been significantly relieved by changing not only what they eat but when they eat. There is enough flexibility in the recommendations below to allow you to fit them into your lifestyle and adopt certain dietary changes in a way that suits you.

How to Change Your Diet

1. Determine your best approach to change. Think of changing the way you eat as though you were removing a Band-Aid. Some people remove theirs millimeter by millimeter, others with one quick rip. There is no right way to do it, but different approaches suit different people. There's going cold turkey or taking it slowly. Know your style and work with it.

2. Acknowledge to yourself that changing your diet is difficult. Food represents more than sustenance. It represents comfort, family, and style of life, reward, deprivation, and ethnicity. Think of how it feels to be away from home and then to return to the food you are used to cooking and eating. Food represents home, what is secure and familiar. None of this is easy to change.

3. Dietary changes can be threatening to others around you. They may need to maintain that the way they eat is really okay. They may want to see you as someone who eats and drinks as they do. We think of people who offer free drugs to others to entice them into using them as deplorable. But have you ever tried telling someone you don't eat sugar anymore? Typical responses are similar to what people who stop drinking alcohol used to hear. "Oh, a little bit won't hurt," or "What's the matter with you!" If you step back for a moment, you may wonder why anyone else should be so threatened by what *you* eat. Why should others care, and if they do, is that your problem or theirs?

4. Try not to fight the change. Think about what you *can* eat and not what you *can't* eat. Make the change a challenge. Adding flavorful, appealing, and healthful foods to your diet is an opportunity to feel better.

5. Give yourself at least three months to see the results of changing the way you eat. Many women with PMS say they have more energy, less anxiety and depression, and fewer headaches after only a few weeks of eating differently, but don't be discouraged if it takes longer.

6. These dietary recommendations aren't effective if you try them only part of the month. You'll have the best results if you incorporate them *all month long,* not just when you are premenstrual. It simply doesn't work to cut down on certain foods that worsen PMS when you are premenstrual.

7. Expect to experience some withdrawal symptoms when you stop ingesting either sugar or caffeine, and expect a period of adjustment to whatever new substances you introduce into your diet. Withdrawal, especially from caffeine, produces lethargy and headaches that peak in about ten days and finally are relieved in about two weeks. Changing the way you eat produces profound differences in how you feel and how you experience yourself.

8. The recommended diet for PMS is similar to but not exactly the same as typical diets for hypoglycemia (low blood sugar).

9. Anything sweet can provoke a lowering of blood sugar, even noncaloric sweeteners. There is evidence that just looking at foods can provoke sugar absorption into cells, and so can just tasting something sweet. Our bodies may respond to look and taste, even when we don't ingest calories.

10. The first and perhaps most important dietary recommendation for women with PMS is to eat more frequently. Going for long periods without food can bring on or intensify symptoms such as tearfulness, anxiety, fatigue, or headache. When you go too long without food, your glucose (blood sugar) level plummets and you become jittery and irritable.

11. How often is "more frequently"? Eating six small meals a day—a snack or meal every two to three hours—will keep your internal furnace burning steadily and evenly. This schedule works well for many women with PMS:

7:00 A.M.	Breakfast
10:00 A.M.	Morning snack
12:30 P.M.	Lunch
3:00 P.M.	Afternoon snack
6:00 P.M.	Dinner
8:30 P.M.	Evening snack

Of course, you can adjust the times of these meals and snacks depending on your schedule. Exactly when you eat meals and snacks is less important than eating regularly, with no more than three hours between meals.

12. *Increase* the amount of complex carbohydrates (as in whole grains and vegetables), lean protein, and lower-fat foods you eat. These foods burn

slowly in the body and, like coal in your internal furnace, provide longer-lasting and continual heat.

13. *Limit* the amount of sugar and caffeine in your daily diet. Eating sweet foods produces a drop in blood sugar and can worsen premenstrual fatigue, depression, headache, anxiety, or other symptoms. Burning sugar (a simple carbohydrate) for fuel is like using newspaper for heat. It burns easily with a bright flame, then quickly dies, and you need more paper. "Limit," of course, is a broad and general term. Some women with PMS find that it works best for them to remove sugar and caffeine from their diets altogether—they often report that it's easier for them not to be "tempted" with even a little coffee, chocolate, et cetera. Others say their PMS symptoms improved when they sharply reduced their intake of caffeine and sweet foods but still allowed themselves that one savored cup of coffee in the morning and the occasional celebratory piece of chocolate. You will be the best judge of what works for you. If giving up sweet foods or caffeine entirely isn't possible for you, make sure you don't have either on an empty stomach and be especially careful about how much sugar or caffeine you have when you are premenstrual.

14. Use alcohol very sparingly, if at all. As both a sugar and a depressant, alcohol can wreak havoc with PMS symptoms. Women are more sensitive to alcohol's effects when they are premenstrual—the same amount of alcohol that made you feel pleasantly relaxed at one time of the month may make you quite intoxicated when you are premenstrual. Some women with PMS crave alcohol premenstrually, seeking the brief sugar "high" or unconsciously using it to "medicate" their symptoms. The same advice applies to alcohol that applies to caffeine and sweets: You can best determine if eliminating it or cutting down on the amount you drink, particularly when you are premenstrual, is the right approach for you.

15. There does not appear to be any reason to limit salt for PMS. Premenstrual bloating is primarily a redistribution of water that takes place whether or not there is increased salt intake. In fact, water retention can be the result of too much sugar—water accumulation blamed on potato chips may actually be from M&M's.

16. The PMS-Management Diet is not a weight-loss diet. Neither losing nor gaining weight will help PMS. Some women are concerned about the

six-small-meals-a-day recommendation—they immediately equate snacking with weight gain. The two don't have to go together—it depends on the choices and quantity of foods you eat. In fact, many women with PMS report that since they began to nourish their bodies regularly during the day they feel more energetic and fit than they have felt in a long time.

17. If reading this much about changing the way you eat has already made you apprehensive, or if you are too depressed to make dietary changes, be kind to yourself; look to other remedies for PMS. Then, as you begin to feel better, you may be able to come back to looking at what you eat.

What Can You Eat?

VEGETABLES: Raw for crisp snacks, sautéed in a little broth or olive oil, or steamed with lemon and pepper, vegetables are good sources of vitamins and fiber and help fill you up without excess fat or calories.

GRAINS, PEAS, BEANS: Eat plenty of whole grains or products made from whole grains. Bread, bagels, tortillas, and cereals made with whole grains are good additions to meals and snacks. Combined with beans or peas, whole grains are excellent protein sources. Soybean products such as tofu and tempeh are high in protein and contain isoflavones. Isoflavones exert a gentle estrogenic effect in the body, which is why soy products are believed to be heart- and bone-enhancing foods.

NUTS AND SEEDS: Nutritious but high in calories, nuts and seeds add flavor and variety to your meals and snacks. A small handful is a good measure, either tossed on your salad or as part of a snack.

FRUITS: Fruit is best when eaten in smaller amounts and in combination with a complex carbohydrate or a protein. Eaten alone, fruit tends to act like candy in the body, producing a temporary rise in blood sugar followed by a sharp drop-off. Enjoy your fruit, but limit it to about three servings a day. (A serving is generally a half cup of fruit or four ounces of juice.)

The following fruits are especially sweet and should be limited to one serving a day. Eating a cup and a half of very sweet fruit defeats the purpose of avoiding sweets.

cherries	*mangoes*
dates	*papayas*
figs	*pineapple*
prunes	*raisins*

DAIRY PRODUCTS: There is no PMS-related reason to avoid dairy products. Lower-fat or nonfat dairy products are good sources of calcium.

LEAN MEAT, POULTRY, AND FISH: Large quantities of animal protein and fat are not particularly healthy. Diets high in animal protein have been linked to breast, colon, and uterine cancer, as well as to heart disease. You don't need to omit meat, poultry, and fish from your diet to improve your PMS symptoms, but you may want to balance your sources of protein, choosing some animal protein and some plant-based protein, like soy products.

WATER: Straight from the tap or in designer bottles, water is one of the most important substances you take into your body. It constitutes the major part of your cellular makeup. Drink water freely. Far from causing bloating, water actually acts as a diuretic. In order for the kidneys to excrete water, they must add salt to it, so drinking plain water leads to excretion of the water plus salt. Premenstrual bloating is a redistribution of water in your body. It is not related to water consumption.

What Should You Avoid?

salty lunch meat, sausage, bacon	*caffeinated drinks, coffee, tea, soda**
high-fat cheeses such as Brie	*artificial sweeteners*
white bread, cake, cookies	*alcohol*
jam, honey, molasses	

How to Use These Food Lists

To enjoy and get the most benefit from the "What Can You Eat" list, combine foods from the different categories whenever you can. Think in terms

---

*Caffeine is also found in chocolate and some over-the-counter cold preparations; read the labels.

of balancing your carbohydrates with a small amount of protein, vegetables, and/or fruit. Here are some examples:

- Brown rice for dinner may sound healthy, but your body will benefit more if you combine it with other foods. Add color, fiber, and energy with vegetables, beans, slivered nuts, or shredded cheese.
- Boost the energy you'll derive from your whole-grain bagel in the morning by spreading it with low-fat or nonfat cream cheese, all-fruit preserves, or unsweetened peanut butter.
- Apples are great snacks—you can keep them in your desk or in your car. Munch on it whole, or cut it in half and pair it with a handful of roasted soy nuts or a slice of low-fat cheese, or dip three or four apple slices in low-fat vanilla yogurt.
- A salad with some protein will give your body more fuel than salad alone. Add sliced hard-boiled eggs, low-fat cheese, lean ham or chicken, or sunflower seeds or other nuts to your greens for more energy.

Your meals can be as elaborate or as simple as you choose. Some women enjoy cooking and experimenting with new foods; others want their meals to be quick and easy. Either of these cooking and eating preferences can be adapted to improve your PMS symptoms, as long as you remember to eat frequently and combine foods.

The Rule of Halves

The PMS-Management Diet isn't based on specific recommendations for *x* grams of protein, fat, and carbohydrates per day. The revised food pyramid, with its emphasis on whole grains, lots of vegetables and fruit, lean protein sources, and more sparing use of fats and sweets, is a good general guideline.

"But how much should I eat?" is a question that comes up often. "What exactly should I have for my meals and snacks?" I generally suggest choosing foods you enjoy from the "What Can You Eat?" list and think in terms of halves. Breakfast can be a half cup of whole-grain cereal with berries and low-fat milk. At your desk or in your car, wherever you find yourself at midmorning, have a handful of whole-grain crackers with carrot or celery sticks or half a banana. At lunchtime, enjoy half a sandwich made with lean turkey on whole-wheat bread and half an apple. Two to three hours later, snack on a half cup of low-fat yogurt or cottage cheese—or the other half of your sandwich—with the rest of your apple. The rule of halves often helps alleviate women's concern that they will be eating too much and gaining weight if they switch their eating patterns to include three meals and three snacks every day.

Avoidance Techniques

Staying away from the "What Should You Avoid?" list poses varying degrees of difficulty for different women. Women with PMS often describe doing well with the PMS-Management Diet until they go on a business trip, to a party, or to dinner at a relative's house, where sweets, alcohol, or other unfriendly foods are in plentiful supply.

These steps for planning and substituting are useful tools to help avoid foods that can worsen PMS symptoms:

- If you're going to a party or a dinner where you aren't sure what will be served, eat a good snack before you go so you won't arrive famished.
- Keep a "survival kit" with you—in the glove compartment of your car, in your desk, or in your carry-on bag if you're traveling. Fill it with foods that will keep, such as whole-grain rice cakes or crackers, nuts, apples, bread sticks, or pretzels.
- In restaurants, check the list of side dishes. You may be able to combine several to create a healthier meal than if you order from the list of entrées.
- When you're eating out, don't hesitate to ask to have something prepared the way you like it: pasta with tomatoes and other vegetables instead of a rich sauce, fish with lemon and herbs and only a very small amount of butter or oil, or pizza with lots of fresh vegetables and herbs and only a very light sprinkling of cheese. Many restaurants are willing to accommodate this type of request.
- If you regularly attend functions where the menu is limited (banquets or fund-raising dinners), mark your calendar to call ahead a couple of days in advance and request a vegetarian plate. Your meal is likely to be healthier and may even be a pleasant change from standard banquet fare.

About Dependence

It's possible to be very dependent on certain foods or drinks for relaxation, stimulation, or comfort. Admittedly, getting rid of this kind of dependence is difficult. The first step is to recognize that you have more than the usual need for a certain food or drink. The best way to recognize this pattern in yourself is to notice your reaction to the idea that you should limit or give something up. If you get anxiety or a sick feeling in your gut, or if you tell yourself you *could* give something up if you *had* to but you're not sure you're ready to, then you're probably hooked.

The second way to know if you are dependent on a food or drink is by actually trying to stop. If you feel worse—depressed or irritable, for example—and believe that some substance will make you feel better, then you have more than the usual reliance on that substance. And you probably will feel better if you consume it, but only temporarily.

If you spend your time fantasizing about a certain food or substance, you need it more than you should. If you dream of candy bars or coffee, your body is probably telling you it is missing them. Most Americans are unable to abstain from coffee or sugar for even a week.

Changing a pattern of dependence on coffee, chocolate, or wine will probably take time, and you can expect to miss these things as you reduce the amount you eat or drink. Remind yourself that the changes you are making are difficult steps toward a long-term goal.

Others may not support your commitment to change the way you eat. They may react with open hostility or subtle attempts to undermine your effort by placing sweets or other foods in view around the house. Children are especially threatened by changes in food. Eating meals together, breaking bread, is a basic part of what we do together as humans, and changes in those patterns can create deep insecurities. For both children and adults, food is often equated with love.

If family, coworkers, or friends challenge or dismiss your efforts to maintain the PMS-Management Diet, it may help to simply say, "I feel much better when I don't eat sweets (drink alcohol, have coffee)," et cetera. Or, if you are under medical care, enlist your doctor as an invisible ally, and say something like, "My doctor recommends that I cut out sweets." You may also want to be candid in asking for support at home or at work: "I'm working hard to change the way I eat so I will feel better; it will help me if I'm not tempted."

> It's wonderful to finally have relief from my depression and moodiness. It's the result of the diet. All symptoms are practically gone except withdrawal, and I can talk myself through because I know I'm premenstrual.

CHAPTER 11

✿

Exercise

Exercise can help provide a sense of well-being as well as an outlet for excess energy, and it is an effective way of relieving body tension. Many women are too fatigued or depressed to exercise when they are premenstrual. Bloating leaves them especially prone to feeling bad about their bodies. It is therefore important to establish an exercise regimen that can be sustained *throughout your menstrual cycle.*

Studies conducted at the University of British Columbia and Kansas State University validated the benefit of exercise for women with PMS, revealing that even moderate exercise reduced symptoms. In the Canadian study, formerly sedentary women who began to run a mile a day reported less breast soreness and bloating after six months. Women in the Kansas State University study reported symptom relief in only three months.

Exercise can become habit-forming and even addictive in a positive sense. Many women find that once they establish a routine of exercise, they feel lost, unsettled, or irritable on days when they cannot continue it. One woman began walking every morning before breakfast. It became her time to be alone, to think, and to move her body. As she realized the importance of her walking, she became better able to protect her time. Looking back, she recalled: "I felt so bad about myself, I didn't think I deserved the time to exercise."

Exercise has two components. One is the physical activity. The other is taking time to care for one's body and one's self. Both are necessary if exercise is to help PMS. Being on your feet all day does not constitute exercise that is beneficial to PMS or to your mood, nor does doing housework or even construction work. Those activities do require movement of the body but without the environment that allows this movement to be translated into a self-nurturing or self-development experience. Doing housework does not decrease depression or lead to an increase in self-esteem, but taking time for a walk, even if the total energy expenditure is less, will combat depression and enhance self-confidence and self-esteem. You must have peace of mind for the exercise to produce its beneficial effects. Aerobic exercise can be fine, but not if you have a two-year-old tugging at your skirt or falling on your stomach. What matters for relief of PMS is not the number of miles walked or jogged but the quality of that experience. The pleasure and benefit of reading books cannot be measured by the number of words read. It is an experience that can only be measured by the enhancement of your sense of well-being.

Exercise must be *pleasurable, daily, at least thirty minutes in duration, and uninterrupted.*

It matters less what the particular exercise is and more that it provides some *pleasure.* If it does not, you will find it almost impossible to be motivated sufficiently to do the exercise when you are premenstrual.

You must strive to exercise daily. The body can come to count on this regular release of tension, and as a result it may begin to store anxieties until that time each day. For women trying to control weight, exercising in the morning leads to more weight loss than exercise done later in the day. Morning exercise seems to set the body's metabolic rate higher so that more calories are burned off during the day.

It is important to differentiate exercise for cardiovascular fitness or weight loss from exercise for PMS. Using stairs instead of elevators will enhance both fitness and weight loss but may do nothing for PMS. It is really the combination of movement and *the sense of well-being* that is helpful for PMS.

Exercises

WALKING: Strolling or race walking both qualify, as well as anything between the two. Walking to work helps for fitness or weight loss but rarely includes the necessary ingredient of peacefulness. As I've stressed, for exercise to help PMS it must include the commitment to take time out for oneself. Taking a walk before the day begins, at lunchtime, after work, or after others come home (to relieve women at home with children) are all ways of releasing tension and moving one's body beneficially. Walking also promotes bone strength, and it can be done in cities and rural areas.

JOGGING: Jogging is a popular form of exercise but, like walking, it may be dependent on weather conditions, except for those people close to an indoor track. Speed isn't important; what does matter is achieving that sense of well-being and then *maintaining* it.

SWIMMING: Swimming is excellent exercise that can be done either outdoors or indoors depending on the time of year and your proximity to pools. For many women it provides a time when they cannot be interrupted as well as an opportunity to move the body. Again, although it would be so much easier if one could prescribe a certain number of laps or miles that would relieve PMS, at issue here, is not the number of laps but rather the quality of the experience.

BIKING AND USING EXERCISE BIKES: The combination of the two, which allows for daily exercise independent of weather, can be exhilarating. Riding an exercise bike can also be boring, but it can be done while reading or listening to music, among other activities.

AEROBIC EXERCISING AND DANCING: This can be done in classes, in front of the TV, with tapes, or with some combination of the above. Few women can or want to go to classes daily, but a combination of classes and home tapes can become a daily routine.

Exercises such as horseback riding, ice-skating, skiing, squash, tennis, volleyball, and others can also be pleasurable and useful. They can be part of your routine, but since they are rarely daily exercises, they should be mixed with others so that you are sure to do something each day.

Planning Exercise

1. Start your exercise program when you are not premenstrual. Take advantage of the good feeling that begins with or shortly after your period

commences. In the midst of PMS not much feels good, so don't expect to implement lifestyle changes then.

2. Give yourself a month or two to establish your regular exercise program. Begin by listing those exercises you might like, those you've always enjoyed, those you didn't enjoy before but might like to try again, those you've always wanted to try but for which you haven't had the time, energy, or motivation.

3. Try different exercises during the first months. For instance, take a long walk one day, swim at a local Y another. If you begin by thinking, "This is what I'm going to have to do each day," you may be defeating yourself at the start. Try jogging one day, not for distance but just to see how it feels. Check TV listings for exercise shows you can watch and participate in at home. Take advantage of health clubs that let you use their facilities once or twice before you have to join.

4. Begin to look at yourself as someone who exercises and is simply looking for the right activity. Imagine yourself dancing, running, or sitting on an exercise bike.

5. If premenstrual fatigue makes it especially hard to motivate yourself to exercise the week before your period, switch to a gentler workout for those days. Yoga and stretching are calming ways to move your body without a jarring effect.

6. Begin an exercise journal. The following pages may be helpful to you in organizing your approach to exercise. Try them, but if keeping such records is stressful, then proceed without them. (See the Appendix on pages 179–80 for additional copies of these forms.)

Exercise Journal

EXERCISE I LIKE	EXERCISE TO RETRY	EXERCISE I ALWAYS WANTED TO TRY

FIVE EXERCISES TO TRY THIS MONTH

1. Exercise _____ How I will do it _____
   _____

2. Exercise _____ How I will do it _____
   _____

3. Exercise _____ How I will do it _____
   _____

4. Exercise _____ How I will do it _____
   _____

5. Exercise _____ How I will do it _____
   _____

FILL-IN EXERCISES While I am trying new forms of exercise I will use the following exercises on a daily basis so that each day I do something.

_____

_____

_____

_____

Weekly Exercise Journal

Use this form to keep track of the exercises you are doing. It will be interesting to see how, over time, your ability and pleasure increase.

Week of _____

	S	M	T	W	T	F	S
EXERCISE							
TIME OF DAY							
HOW LONG							
HOW IT FELT							
WHAT NEEDS TO BE CHANGED							

CHAPTER 12

❀

Stress Management
and PMS

"The Body Takes on the Pain of the Soul"

Stress does not cause PMS, but it can add to premenstrual symptoms and to premenstrual magnification of symptoms. PMS, however, can be a cause of stress.

What is stress? It is a state of tension with both emotional and physiological manifestations. The body's response to stress is to stimulate the hypothalamus (the "conductor" of PMS) and to alter brain-wave activity. Feeling stressed or having a physical reaction to stress is not an act of conscious will. It is a physiological and chemical alteration of the brain affecting the hypothalamus, which integrates and mediates neurological and endocrine responses. Since this area already appears to be dysfunctional in PMS, the addition of stress stimuli can make the symptoms worse. On an emotional level, the combination of *constant stress* and PMS, in which there is often an inner pull toward quiet or even withdrawal, add to the confusion, tension, and occasional panic of the syndrome.

So what do you do? The first thing to do is to identify areas of major stress. People are often afraid to acknowledge stressful situations because they fear that they are then supposed to give them up, but this is not necessarily so. Some stresses are useful. When not incapacitating, stress can lead to increased performance and creativity. Without deadlines, for example, we would all probably accomplish little. And stress can be an important component in challenge. The object is not necessarily to give up stress but to have some control over it and to be able to choose which stresses to handle and which to let go of. Some stresses we may not be able to do anything about at this time in our lives, but even coming to terms with that reality can be helpful.

Looking at Stress

Stress can arise from any of the following sources. It can be useful to look at each and ask yourself these questions:

1. Work:
   What is the work I am doing?
   Do I enjoy it?
   Would I rather be doing something else?
   How important is that something else to me?

2. Health:
   Do I have health problems other than my PMS?
   Am I satisfied with my body?
   Am I at war with my body?
   What would I like to change?
   What do I think I might be able to change?

3. Personal Finance:
   Am I satisfied with my present financial life?
   Is it different from the circumstances of my childhood?
   Is there a disparity of financial goals within my home?
   Do I have control over my financial situation?
   Am I comfortable with the way in which money is handled in my life?

4. Primary adult relationships:
   What are my primary relationships like, with my husband, lover,
   *   partner, parent, friends?*
   What are the difficult areas?

What is most gratifying?
For the moment, am I basically satisfied in each relationship?

5. Children: Children themselves can cause stress, and so can the work
    involved in caring for them. Added to that is the stress women feel
    in protecting their children from their own premenstrual mood
    swings and anger.
    What are the good and the difficult times with my children?
    Do I feel alone? Supported?
    Do I think they are difficult children?
    Do I think I am difficult as a parent?
    What do I need to make my life with them better?
    *Am I in conflict with others about the children—that is, with spouse,
        parents, friends?*

6. Friendships:
    Do I have a network of supportive friends?
    Has the network changed recently? Have I isolated myself?
    Have I filled my life with friends to avoid being alone?

7. Self:
    Am I comfortable with myself when I'm not in the midst of PMS?
    What pleases me about myself?
    What might I wish to change?

8. Time:
    How do I relate to the concept of time?
    *Does the word time make me panic because there never seems to be
        enough?*
    Which of my time stresses seem temporary?
    Which seem to be a permanent part of my life?
    How would I like to change my relationship to time?

9. Being alone:
    Do I have time alone?
    Am I afraid to be alone?
    Is there support for me to have time alone?
    Do I believe I deserve it?

10. Spirituality:
    What are my present beliefs?

Have they changed?
Am I satisfied with changes in my sense of spirituality?
Is there conflict in my family regarding spirituality?
Do I give room to this part of my life?
How is my spirituality affected by PMS?

> *I consider myself a very religious person. One of the worst parts about having PMS has been that I sometimes lose my faith when I am in the worst PMS. I can't find anything to believe in. I'm just miserable, and I want to get angry with God. I try to look at what I am supposed to learn and why I am suffering, but I can't find any meaning in it, except that I understand other people's pain more.*

At times, PMS occurs in a woman's life when she is undergoing deep questioning of her identity, purpose, and belief systems. The crisis of body dysfunction accompanies the crisis of being. I have watched them develop together and have seen them resolve themselves simultaneously.

Methods of Stress Reduction

Stress reduction requires you to recognize that stress exists and then that you desire to lessen it. There is a high that comes with stressful living, as well as a high associated with living from crisis to crisis. Trying to reduce stress without recognizing this can lead to failure. The intent to lessen stress is helpful in itself, but looking for the perfect way to do it or expecting to become stress-free in a week can create even more stress.

Reducing stress is more than learning to forget it or to stop getting so upset. Few of us are free of the voices in our heads that constantly give us instructions. What is required here is a more profound alteration in your way of being, a shift in how you experience yourself and your environment. Achieving that goal is not easy.

Relaxation and stress reduction do not happen by trying harder to make them happen. What is needed is the opposite of learning a language—where the more you practice, the more you learn. Here the harder you try to relax, the less you are going to succeed.

It is important to look at stress reduction as a "one day at a time" process. There is always stress, there are always stressful events, but recognizing what is outside yourself versus what is within your own control makes PMS, as well as much of life, easier. Stress reduction is not something one simply does daily for a particular amount of time. It is a way of approaching one's life. It's like a shift in background color of a painting, or a change in a camera lens. It is the creation of a new way of experiencing yourself and the world.

Stress-reduction techniques (a long phrase for what is supposed to make life easier) are most useful if they become integrated into your life on a regular basis. Unlike exercises that demand a separate time, these methods can often be done in ten-minute intervals—at work, at the end of a long line at the bank, or even in the midst of a traffic jam—when remembering to focus or release or just to relax your muscles can have a tremendously beneficial effect on your sense of peace.

Try to schedule a regular time (however brief) each day in which to practice some of these methods. Post reminders to yourself in strategic places (on your mirror or on the refrigerator door, for example) to use the techniques. Most important, though, is to recognize that inner change does not occur overnight, and it rarely happens in an even, steady progression.

Begin to try out various ways of reducing stress. There are many magazine articles, books, and cassette programs about stress reduction, as well as classes offered at schools, Y's, and other places.

Look at the following suggestions for ways to reduce stress, live with them, think about them, try them, but most of all, let yourself begin to see yourself as a person who will be living with *less stress.* That's not to say that life will go easily, but the aim is to experience stresses without being eaten up inside or lashing out at others.

A Word About These Methods

They seem simple: *Find a quiet place . . . breathe . . . meditate . . . let go . . . imagine a peaceful scene . . .* but, they are not. As with diet, one doesn't change a lifetime of patterning in a day. Presented below is information about some of these methods to give you an idea of what they are like so you can further pursue those that appeal to you.

As you begin to learn these methods, you need to make room for them in your life, as well as for the changes they will create. Learn several ways of using these techniques, when you might *not* want to use them, and what to do when they don't seem to be working. Some people become anxious when they begin to try these new things. Don't give up, but also don't force yourself.

MEDITATION: Many forms of meditation can help induce a sense of inner peace and an increased ability to deal with stressful situations. Meditation is a simple mental technique that allows the mind to calm down. It has, at times, been associated with religious and cultic activities, but there are methods of meditating that anyone can learn easily and that require no affinity to a group or belief system. Meditation simply consists of creating quiet time in which to sit or walk alone and then silently repeating a soothing sound or word in a special manner or simply paying attention to breathing. Some people can meditate while swimming or jogging.

RELEASING, FOCUSING: These two methods of dealing with one's own hair-trigger reaction to stress can be useful for PMS. They consist of simple techniques for teaching oneself to let go of overinvolvement in the outcome of a particular problem in order to cope more calmly and effectively. Again, the object is not to float into nirvana at the sign of stressful events or to drop out but rather to learn ways in which you can peacefully and with satisfaction survive some of the unavoidable stress and chaos of life.

SELF-HYPNOSIS: This is a process of self-suggestion one can learn either from a clinical hypnotist and/or from reading books about the subject. It is especially useful for reducing stress, breaking habits, and dealing with cravings.

RELAXATION TECHNIQUES: These are methods of directly relaxing the body. They can be done by concentrating on breathing, by attending progressively to body muscles and their tension or relaxation, or by imagining peaceful scenes, a process often called visualizing (or imagining). There are many varieties of these techniques. Read about them, and try what seems appealing to you.

YOGA: Yoga involves both breathing and stretching exercises, which many people find relaxing. There are several books and videotapes that can be useful for someone trying yoga alone, and many communities have responsible yoga classes. There are also yoga classes on TV, usually early in the morning or late at night. Yoga exercises can put undue strain on the body, so it is important to proceed slowly.

MASSAGE: Regular massage, especially during the premenstrual period, may provide physical relaxation, which in turn reduces emotional tension and thus lessens stress reactions. I sometimes think of PMS as a brick wall that must be broken through each month for a woman to feel relief. Some force is necessary to overcome the emotional state, and that force can be medication, a bout of tears, an angry outburst, or a good massage.

EXPRESSIVE ARTS: Drawing, music, writing, knitting, needlework, and baking bread can all give you a sense of peace that goes beyond the moment and affects general mood and coping ability.

JOURNAL WRITING: Keeping a journal requires some privacy and some time to oneself. There are many ways of using this technique. It can simply represent a way of silently screaming at what bothers you, or it can include a process of thinking "out loud" but alone. It also provides an ongoing record for looking back as you begin to take hold of your PMS and your life in general; and it can be an expression of your fantasy and of longings. All these uses are healthy and can lead to the reduction of stress. Here are some ways to start a journal. As with exercise, the form often matters less than what it comes to mean to you as an experience.

- Use a blank book, preferably one that you find appealing.
- Try using a dated journal. The dates on each page can be an impetus to write, but they can also be oppressive, so watch your own reaction and modify your journal writing accordingly.
- Be flexible about what you want to cover each day. For example, your journal can describe your emotions, your exercise, the food you are eating, stresses, feelings about relationships, work, time, aspirations, resentments, support (present or absent), what you are doing for yourself today, what you are learning about yourself at this time.
- Go back to your journal when you are not premenstrual, and reassess your feelings, reactions, what you were doing for or against yourself. The "Bad Day Report" at the end of this chapter (page 114) can be useful. Use it to record the events of a particularly stressful day so you can analyze it more closely. Date it and note the day of your last period. You will want

to know if this bad day was premenstrual or not. Describe the day, and then a week or so later go back and see if it now looks different. What can you learn now about the stress, your reaction to it, or your PMS?

Under stress it is easy to forget everything you know about coping mechanisms. Stress reactions can interfere with good judgment, and at those moments when life seems out of control, you may not remember your stress-reduction techniques. In spite of all your reading and efforts, you may have setbacks at times of crisis. The next crisis, though, may be a bit easier because of what you have learned. And the next easier still.

Bad Day Report

DATE _____ LAST PERIOD _____

DAY OF CYCLE _____

What happened?

Foods eaten (note also any long stretches without eating):

Exercise:

Current stresses:

Review of the day several days later: How does the day look in retrospect? Were issues raised that still may be important? Was your diet that day a healthy one? What have you learned?

CHAPTER 13

❋

Vitamins and Nonprescription PMS Remedies

PMS Vitamins

Many PMS vitamin formulations are now available. Some, like Optivite and ProCycle, consist of formulations that have been shown to be effective in clinical research and have been used successfully in tens of thousands of women for more than a decade. The development of PMS products is a dramatic change from the days when women with PMS were cavalierly told to take remedies intended for menstrual cramps but that did nothing to relieve their PMS.

The proper vitamin preparation should be an integral component of your self-care program to manage PMS, but it's important to choose products carefully. Keep these guidelines in mind as you consider over-the-counter PMS products, and always keep your doctor informed of any vitamins and supplements you take—even over-the-counter ones.

How to Take a PMS Vitamin

It's important to take a PMS supplement all month long, not just when you are premenstrual. Don't expect immediate symptom relief—it may take two to three months to realize the benefits.

If you are taking additional calcium, more than is contained in your PMS supplement, it is best to separate the doses. Take your PMS supplement in the morning and your calcium in the evening.

Vitamin B$_6$

Formulas for PMS generally contain amounts of the B vitamins and magnesium that are higher than the recommended daily allowance. Some studies show that vitamin B$_6$, when taken as part of a B-complex vitamin that also contains magnesium, is helpful in relieving certain PMS symptoms, especially bloating, depression, fluid retention, food cravings, and fatigue.

The usual dosage of B$_6$ for PMS is up to 300 milligrams per day. The B-complex vitamins work together and should not be taken individually. Vitamin B$_6$ alone, taken in very high dosages—over 2,000 milligrams per day—and without other B vitamins and magnesium, can produce serious side effects—even irreversible nerve damage. Undesirable side effects of B$_6$ include headache, dizziness, nausea, and restless sleep or nightmares. If you develop these symptoms, discontinue the B$_6$ and consult your physician. You should take B$_6$ with food to avoid stomach upset.

Calcium and Magnesium

The correct use of magnesium and calcium for PMS can be quite confusing. There is evidence that women with PMS need more magnesium than is found in standard multivitamins, which contain a two-to-one ratio of calcium to magnesium. Women with PMS benefit from *reversing* this ratio—two times the amount of magnesium to calcium (250 milligrams magnesium to 125 milligrams of calcium). However, women with PMS who also have menstrual cramping should take the higher ratio of calcium during menstruation. The situation becomes even more complicated as we also become aware of the need for extra calcium to prevent osteoporosis.

Supplements are available that contain a balanced combination of B vitamins, magnesium, and calcium and that have a reliable track record in helping to manage PMS symptoms. Be sure to compare ingredients and price before you buy a PMS supplement.

Oil of Evening Primrose

The evening primrose is a North American wildflower whose seeds contain an oil that has been found helpful in PMS. The oil contains an essential fatty acid, gamma-linolenic acid, which, incidentally, is also found in human breast milk. Several studies have shown oil of evening primrose to be effective for physical symptoms of PMS, especially for breast tenderness and swelling. In some cases it has also benefited the emotional symptoms.

The recommended dosage of oil of evening primrose is two 500-milligram capsules, taken twice daily (2,000 milligrams per day). As with all supplements, check with your doctor before taking this.

Oil of evening primrose is best absorbed when taken with a B-complex vitamin and at least 600 milligrams of vitamin C per day. It is also a good idea to take it after eating to avoid stomach upset.

The preparation is available without prescription and is widely sold in pharmacies and health-food stores. Some products contain *other* non-effective oils rather than genuine oil of evening primrose, so be sure to read labels carefully.

Antiprostaglandins

Prostaglandins are a group of hormones that help to regulate the contractions of muscles in some internal organs. Antiprostaglandins inhibit contractions.

Antiprostaglandins are administered orally, as pills, when symptoms are present. The most common side effects are gastrointestinal irritation, with nausea, gas, or diarrhea.

Premenstrual physical symptoms such as cramps, headaches, bloating, nausea, or breast pain are sometimes responsive to antiprostaglandin medications. Some of the more common agents with antiprostaglandin activity are aspirin, ibuprofen, naproxen, and mefenamic acid.

Herbal Approaches

Herbs have been used for healing since antiquity and remain a major treatment for illness in many parts of the world today. They are an integral part of many cultures—in highly industrialized parts of the world as well as in the developing countries. Herbs at times have been the antecedents of current pharmaceuticals.

Crushed, dried, ground into powder, or steeped as tea, herbs have been used by women for thousands of years to ease labor pains or menstrual cramps, stimulate lactation, induce relaxation, fight fevers and infections—essentially in all areas of health. Americans are now using herbs in record numbers, trying to prevent, cure, or alleviate the pain of chronic conditions that may not or have not responded to other treatments.

We are entering a time of rapid change in our approach to herbal therapies, which are increasingly being accepted within mainstream health care. Research is beginning to shed light on how some of them work, and on ones that do not work. Herbs present a dilemma. Their widespread use throughout the world and throughout history suggests their effectiveness. However, they have not been subjected to the rigors of research that we have come to expect of pharmaceutical agents we use. Herbal preparations are not subjected to the same level of standardization and quality control as regulated medicines. Dosages may vary from preparation to preparation. *Natural* does not necessarily mean safe.

Recent research has begun to differentiate among some of the effective herbs and their methods of action. New scientific data will provide reassurance to the health care community, as well as create opportunities for more standardized products. Ultimately, we want to have safe products that we can trust to be effective.

For the present time, you must exercise caution when using herbal preparations (as you should with all medications). Health care providers are increasingly open to discussing herbal treatments. You should find a provider whom you can trust to give you guidance, and always report any side effects immediately.

DONG QUAI (ANGELICA SINENSIS): This herb, which is often used for PMS, is a phytoestrogen, a plant with mild estrogenic effects in the body. Taken alone or as part of a treatment program that includes acupuncture, dong quai is reported to be useful in balancing a woman's ratio of estrogen and progesterone. The theory is that dong quai has an equal ability to stimulate or dampen estrogen's effects. In other words, when estrogen is low, dong quai corrects the hormone balance by exerting a gentle estrogenic effect. If there is too much estrogen in the body, dong quai is believed to occupy estrogen-receptor sites, thereby balancing the estrogen/progesterone ratio. The European variety of dong quai is called angelica.

Dong quai can be taken as a powdered root or tea or as a fluid extract. Dosages vary by the type and quality of the preparation. You should consult with a health care practitioner about dosage, because it will depend on the particular preparation.

SAINT-JOHN'S-WORT: Saint-John's-wort *(Hypericum perforatum)* has a rich folk history of use in treating wounds, of inspiring a saint's benediction, and in protecting its users from danger. Saint-John's-wort is being evaluated in this country as a potential treatment for depression.

As an extract from the perennial plant, the active ingredient in Saint-John's-wort is hypericin. In the brain, hypericin may prolong the effects of the brain chemical serotonin, which presumably would have a positive effect on mood.

Women may try Saint-John's-wort to help with depression for several reasons: because standard antidepressant medication has not helped them; they prefer to try a nonprescription remedy first; or they have experienced unpleasant side effects from antidepressant medication (dry mouth, constipation, insomnia, or diminished sex drive).

Saint-John's-wort now appears to have some promise in alleviating mild to moderate depression. There is no evidence yet to suggest that severely depressed individuals will be helped by this herb. If you are already taking prescription antidepressants, never stop taking them to take Saint-John's-wort before checking with your doctor.

There are also no data suggesting that Saint-John's-wort addresses depression associated with PMS. However, women who are depressed throughout the month and who find that their depression is magnified during their premenstrual phase may consider Saint-John's-wort among their options.

As with all herbal preparations, the quality of the product varies greatly. You should never begin any herbal treatments while on antidepressant therapies because of the danger of drug interactions. If you are on antide-pressants, you must work with your physician to taper your medication gradually while monitoring the effectiveness of the herbal preparation. It can take months for Saint-John's-wort to become effective.

PMS Teas and Other Beverages

Several PMS teas are available. While no clinical evidence demonstrates that the herbs in these teas will improve PMS symptoms, it may be that the self-nurturing act of stopping to have a cup of tea can itself reduce stress and improve a sense of well-being. And there may be active ingredients we just haven't identified yet. This is another area that will change rapidly in the next few years.

PMS beverages containing carbohydrates, vitamins, and minerals may help to minimize symptoms by affecting serotonin. A snack of complex carbohydrates combined with a small amount of protein will probably achieve this effect as well.

Finally, never assume that because something is sold without a pre-scription that it is safe in any quantity. Don't exceed the recommended dosage of a nutritional supplement or other over-the-counter product. And, just as you would with any other product you buy, evaluate claims about effectiveness carefully. Nothing, unfortunately, is a quick fix or silver bullet for PMS. It's important to remember that a self-care program for managing PMS symptoms is most successful when it combines eating well, regular exercise, stress reduction, and nutritional supplements as needed.

CHAPTER 14

✿

Progesterone

I was living a nightmare, ashamed of myself because of the way I was acting. But I couldn't help it. I would hide in my room, yell, and hit out at my husband. I tried to kill myself twice. Now that I have been taking progesterone I have not had any problems for two years. I feel normal again.

The difference between the way I feel now since I have been taking natural progesterone is very simple: It's like night and day.

Progesterone is not a self-help treatment, but I discuss it here for four reasons.

1. There are women for whom self-help methods like eating well, exercising regularly, nutritional supplements, and stress reduction are simply not enough to manage their symptoms.

2. Women may do very well for years managing their symptoms with self-care and then find, as they reach their late thirties or early forties, that their symptoms intensify and seem not to respond as well as they once did to self-care.

3. Some women's lives are so difficult or stressed that they simply cannot manage a PMS self-help program. They need the most relief with the least investment of time.

4. Natural-progesterone therapy for PMS is still not well understood among many medical practitioners and patients. It's essential that a woman considering its use learn what this therapy involves, how to use it, and what to expect, so that she can discuss it with her provider.

Progesterone remains a mainstay of PMS treatment. Research results have varied, with some studies showing effectiveness, and others not. But research conditions can be very different from those of clinical practice. Equally important has been the relative lack of side effects experienced when this medication is given properly.

People do not always react identically to medications. This is especially true of women and hormonal preparations. Therefore, you may have an unexpected response. Some women are fine taking the hormonal preparations that are used for birth control or hormone replacement therapy. Other women may become mildly depressed. Some women report that taking estrogen makes them feel wonderful. It is essential that you pay attention to how you feel on any new medication, and not try to fit your response to what you are expecting.

Earlier in this book I talked about medicine becoming increasingly responsive to women's experiences. This will continue to happen only if women tell their health care providers how they are really feeling and their health care providers listen to them!

History

Progesterone therapy for PMS was suggested in the late 1940s, primarily by Dr. Katharina Dalton in England. Its use in the United States began in the very late 1970s and early 1980s following sensationalistic reports on PMS in the British press. In the United States, progesterone was compounded by individual pharmacists in response to women who were seeking help for PMS, a newly recognized condition.

Two pharmacists in Madison, Wisconsin, began compounding progesterone preparations and started what later became PMS Access, a national hotline for women with PMS and a source of physician training, medication, and educational materials and programs. At the same time, clinics and programs sprang up in Massachusetts, Utah, California, New York, and North Carolina. Women, and their physicians, were increasingly able to obtain reliable treatment and information.

After nearly two decades, tens of thousands of women have used natural-progesterone therapy for PMS with good results. In spite of these numbers, confusion still exists about this treatment for PMS.

The Hormone

Progesterone is produced by the ovaries every month from Day 14 until Day 28 of the menstrual cycle, when your period begins. This progesterone prepares the lining of the uterus for a fertilized egg. Progesterone is the hormone of pregnancy and means, literally, "for gestation." If fertilization and implantation do not occur, your progesterone level falls and a new cycle begins.

In a monthly pattern, progesterone gradually rises starting around Day 14, peaking around Day 21, and falling gradually until Day 28, when menstruation begins. (Your ovaries do not produce progesterone during the first half of your menstrual cycle.) After ovulation, progesterone gradually rises. If you become pregnant, the placenta produces progesterone in amounts thirty to fifty times higher than those found in the nonpregnant state. If you are not pregnant, cyclic production of progesterone continues.

Progesterone has a calming effect on some women. High progesterone levels may be one reason some women report feeling especially well during pregnancy. Some women even use expressions like "cloud nine," or say they would not mind staying pregnant, or that they look forward to another pregnancy because they feel so well.

The Medication

Progesterone is prescribed by a physician for a woman during the second half of her menstrual cycle. It's very important to distinguish between natural progesterone, a prescription medication that is identical to the hormone your ovaries produce, and synthetic progestin.

Synthetic progestins, such as those found in oral contraceptives, are similar to but not identical to the hormones produced naturally in the body. They may actually suppress your body's output of the natural hormone. Some synthetic progestins may intensify, rather than relieve, PMS symptoms.

Natural progesterone and synthetic progestins act very differently in the body and cannot be used interchangeably. Unfortunately, confusion between the two persists, so it's very important to verify exactly what is prescribed if you are given a prescription for progesterone.

What Natural Progesterone Isn't

The molecular structure of natural progesterone, not the *source* of progesterone, is what distinguishes natural progesterone from the synthetic progestins. Some people mistakenly assume that "natural" progesterone is an herbal or organic substance, something you would buy in a health-food store. It isn't. Natural progesterone (progesterone USP) is a highly purified, quality pharmaceutical preparation primarily derived from the soy plant. It is a prescription medication that can be individually compounded by a pharmacist in various forms. Natural progesterone is also commercially made by major pharmaceutical manufacturers and regulated by the Food and Drug Administration (FDA).

When to Take Natural Progesterone

Most often, natural progesterone is prescribed to be taken during the second half of the menstrual cycle, from ovulation until menstruation begins. Some women with PMS use progesterone only during their difficult cycles, not every month. Many use it for just a few days before menstruation. You can stop progesterone therapy at the end of any cycle. Most women do not need to withdraw or taper off the medication slowly; check with your doctor.

How to Take It

Natural progesterone is available in many different forms. Deciding which one is best for you depends on several factors:

- Ease of absorption—how much of the medication gets into your blood-stream, how fast, and how long it lasts
- Ease of administration—how easy the medication is to take
- Cost

The most commonly prescribed forms of natural progesterone are:

ORAL: Micronized progesterone can be taken orally in capsule or tablet form. (*Micronized* means broken down into very tiny particles.) Women with PMS report best results when using the long-acting oral tablet, an even-release form that can be taken twice a day to produce consistent levels of the medication in the body throughout the day, which is important.

SUPPOSITORIES: Natural-progesterone suppositories can be administered rectally or vaginally. They provide consistent absorption rates. Some women may experience vaginal leakage as the suppository melts. Rectal suppositories can also stimulate the bowel.

RECTAL SUSPENSION: Natural progesterone is suspended in water and administered rectally using a small syringe with applicator. Advantages of this form include the fact that it is easy to adjust the dosage level, it has few side effects, and it is among the least expensive forms of the medication. This method of administration was the first one developed in the United States.

TRANSDERMAL CREAM, GEL, OR LOTION: Progesterone cream, gel, or lotion is best absorbed when applied to the skin on the hands, but it can also be applied to the skin on the stomach, thighs, or inner arms, one to two times a day. Advantages of the transdermal form include ease of use and the fact that low dosages produce symptom relief. A disadvantage is that it is easy to inadvertently keep increasing the dose, or "try a bit more."

SUBLINGUAL: Progesterone can be compounded into sublingual tablets that are placed under the tongue to dissolve. This dosage form tends to produce a "roller-coaster" effect in many women.

INJECTION: Injectable progesterone is available, although it has a somewhat limited therapeutic use. Injections are especially good for immediate relief of the most acute symptoms or as a diagnostic tool. The medication is injected deep into the muscle, which may cause pain and irritation. Injections are normally given at least once a day or every other day. Since the development of oral preparations and of gels, injection as a route of administration is unusual.

Natural-Progesterone Dosage Ranges

The chart below shows common dosage ranges. These are only guidelines to follow in consultation with your health care provider. Management of PMS, whether by self-help or medication, still requires tailoring the regimen depending upon the symptoms.

FORM	AMOUNT	FREQUENCY
Oral micronized capsule	100 milligrams	2 to 4 times daily
Even-release tablet	200–300 milligrams	2 times daily
Suppositories	200–400 milligrams	2 times daily
Suspension	200–400 milligrams	2 times daily
Cream, gel, or lotion	10–30 milligrams	2 times daily
Injection	50–100 milligrams	Daily or every other day

What to Expect

Most women tolerate natural progesterone well. Infrequent side effects may include:

- Drowsiness or dizziness with the oral form. If drowsiness or dizziness occur, the dosage may be too high and need to be reduced. Taking natural progesterone with food also helps to avoid drowsiness.
- Delay in the onset of the menstrual period. If this happens and your period is more than a day or two late, you may need to stop taking progesterone to bring on your period, then resume taking it fourteen days after your period starts.
- Slight flushing. This is normal, because progesterone may raise your body temperature about a degree.

Caution About Wild-Yam Cream

Many wild-yam creams marketed as PMS-relief products contain little or no progesterone and are very expensive. Their labels may contain terms like "balancing formula" or "progesterone precursor." Wild-yam cream and natural-progesterone cream are not the same. If a wild-yam cream contains natural progesterone, it is because the manufacturer has added progesterone USP, the prescription medication, to it. Wild yams themselves do not contain progesterone, and your body doesn't convert wild-yam extract into progesterone.

If the amount of progesterone in a product is below 0.016 percent (less than 5 milligrams per 30 grams), the product can be marketed as an over-the-counter, or OTC, preparation. The amount of progesterone in wild-yam creams varies greatly—from none at all to as high as 10 percent. It's often difficult to ascertain exactly how much, if any, natural progesterone a wild-yam or other over-the-counter PMS cream contains.

A better option is to have your doctor write a prescription for progesterone. That prescription will then be compounded—formulated just for you—by a registered pharmacist. A prescription progesterone cream will often be less expensive than wild-yam cream or an over-the-counter progesterone cream. Most important, you and your doctor will know exactly how much progesterone you're getting. Your doctor can adjust the progesterone dosage in the cream based on your response. Many insurance companies will reimburse the cost of prescription progesterone cream.

Do I Need Natural Progesterone?

Some women choose to try natural-progesterone therapy right away because they are seeking immediate relief from their symptoms. They often feel that the time needed to adjust diet, exercise, and stress-reduction patterns is something they cannot manage. Natural progesterone often does provide relief very quickly, within an hour.

Other women prefer to have their progesterone levels measured before taking a prescription hormone, but there is no conclusive diagnostic test to determine if a woman has PMS. New tests are being developed, though, to give more accurate information about hormone levels, particularly progesterone.

Is Natural Progesterone FDA-Approved?

The Food and Drug Administration (FDA) serves several functions with respect to medications. The first is the approval of medications for specific uses or illnesses (the indications for use) based upon the safety of the drug, and establishing that it works for that indication (efficacy). The FDA also approves the specific wording for marketing that can be used on labels or in advertising for the drugs and indications it has approved. For instance, when you see an advertisement on TV for a pain medication, the FDA has determined what can be said and what claims the manufacturer can make. The FDA does not, however, regulate physicians' practices. Physicians can make a professional judgment to use any drug when deemed the best choice for the treatment of a patient. Therefore, a physician can prescribe progesterone for PMS, even if the FDA has not approved that indication for its use. This practice, which is known as "off-label" prescribing, is commonplace.

Progesterone has been approved for use in assisted-reproductive technology to ensure implantation of the embryo. It has also been approved to induce menstruation in the case of secondary amenorrhea (that is, missed menstrual periods in a woman who has at some time menstruated). In the case of progesterone, the manufacturer has demonstrated to the FDA that it is safe to use and of benefit in those conditions. However, a physician can prescribe progesterone for PMS, just as a physician can prescribe other medications that do not have FDA approval specifically for use in PMS.

Research in PMS is still relatively new, and there will eventually be new products approved for its treatment. It is also possible that a PMS indication for progesterone will be approved in the future.

A critical function of the FDA is the regulation of the development and manufacturing of the actual preparations used. In that regard, the FDA allows the sale of products contingent on their having been developed and manufactured according to FDA guidelines, referred to as Good Manufacturing Practice, or GMP's. These drug regulations insure the quality standards of the medications that are sold. Therefore, in order to be sold in the United States, the progesterone has to have been manufactured according to these FDA standards.

Studies

Clinical studies on the effectiveness of progesterone therapy for PMS shows mixed results, at least in part because of significant methodological problems in the studies.

- There is no uniform definition of what constitutes PMS.
- Treatment schedules have varied from study to study.
- Progesterone dosages have varied from study to study.
- Results by one researcher have not been reproducible by the next.
- The women in the studies may be quite different from the general population of women with PMS.

Conclusions

Natural progesterone has been effective for many women in relieving their premenstrual symptoms. The percentages and efficacy rates are still not clear.

If you are considering natural-progesterone therapy for PMS, read all you can. Identify your issues and concerns and discuss them with your doctor. Recognize too that you can change your decisions about treatment. Flexibility, patience with the treatment process, and compassion for oneself are the most important elements in designing your course of treatment.

CHAPTER 15

❀

Other Prescription Treatments for PMS

Antidepressants

> *Years ago I suffered from severe depression. I was hospitalized several times, and it was always premenstrually. The antidepressants did nothing for the premenstrual depressions. Now I'm on antidepressants that work premenstrually as well as the rest of the month.*

Antidepressant therapy has changed dramatically in the past ten years. Prior to the development of the newer serotonin-increasing medications, antidepressants were often effective for the underlying state of depression but did little for the premenstrual magnification of depression. Women would feel improved and then premenstrually find themselves once again depressed. In addition, the earlier antidepressants had more intrusive side effects than the recent drugs.

The distinction between PMS and depression is clouded by the current widespread use of antidepressants. Antidepressants may improve the mood of people whether they are depressed or not.

As described in earlier chapters, the distinction is further blurred by research methods that didn't always separate PMS from conditions of depression or anxiety. Much of the research was conducted on women who had premenstrual magnification of underlying depression. Therefore, since the women in the studies may have had depression, it is not surprising that their moods were improved by the use of antidepressants. Establishing a clear diagnosis is critical in deciding upon the correct treatment.

A group of antidepressants, the selective serotonin reuptake inhibitors (SSRI's), are commonly prescribed for PMS as well as for depression and premenstrual magnification of depression. This group of compounds acts by increasing the available amount of serotonin, the brain chemical thought to regulate mood. Common generic agents are paroxetine, fluoxetine, sertraline, and fluvoxamine. These medications take days to weeks before they are effective. However, new ones are rapidly being developed that are expected to take effect much more quickly.

These medications may be useful if depressive symptoms do not respond to dietary changes or other treatment options such as natural-progesterone supplementation.

Some women are under the mistaken impression that they can take these antidepressants intermittently—either for part of the month or only during those months when they are having difficult symptoms. However, these antidepressants should not be used in that manner and need to be tapered slowly when they are discontinued. Stopping abruptly or taking them sporadically can produce unpleasant side effects such as dizziness, sleep disturbances, agitation, irritability, or confusion. The consequences can be even more serious if a person who is severely depressed discontinues medication abruptly.

The symptoms resulting from discontinuation of antidepressants—aches and pains and extreme lethargy—may resemble other illnesses such as flu. The symptoms may be misinterpreted as a worsening of anxiety or depression, with subsequent unnecessary increase in medication.

Many other psychotherapeutic agents are prescribed for depression and anxiety that may be influenced by the menstrual cycle. They fall into the following categories:

TRICYCLICS: All of these drugs, which include amitriptyline, nortriptyline, doxepin, imipramine, and protriptyline, are somewhat sedating. Major side effects are constipation, dry mouth, blurred vision, gastrointestinal difficulties, heart palpitations and irregularities, difficulty reaching orgasm, weight gain, urinary retention, and orthostatic hypotension (where getting up suddenly produces a drop in blood pressure and subsequent faintness). Antidepressants tend to interact with other medications, so you should always check with a doctor before combining antidepressant therapy with any other medications. All antidepressants work only when they reach a certain blood level over a period of time. Therefore results are usually not seen in less than two to three weeks. Discontinuation should never be abrupt and should be done only under medical supervision. The effects of stopping medication may not be clear for two to three weeks.

MAO INHIBITORS: Phenelzine and tranylcypromine are the most commonly prescribed MAO (monoamine oxidase) inhibitors. These drugs are considered stronger antidepressants than tricyclics, and in addition to having the same general side effects, they can also in rare cases produce agitation, confusion, and hallucinations. They react much more strongly with other medications and with certain foods. Taking an MAO inhibitor requires adhering to a very strict diet from which many common and nutritious foods such as cheese, chicken liver, yeast, and citrus fruits must be omitted.

LITHIUM SALTS: This medication, which has been in and out of favor over the years, is currently used for manic-depressive illness, now called bipolar disorder. While it appears quite effective in controlling the excitable (manic) phase of the manic-depressive cycle, it requires frequent monitoring of the patient's blood to protect against possible adverse changes in blood chemistry. In general, it is not prescribed for depression alone without careful consideration of its side effects, particularly since its effectiveness for depression is still controversial. While both manic-depressive illness and PMS are cyclic, it is PMS that is tied to the menstrual cycle.

ANXIOLYTICS: These are antianxiety medications that tend to calm states of anxiety or agitation. The most common ones used today are alprazolam, oxazepam, diazepam, and chlordiazepoxide. They used to be called tranquilizers.

Cycle-Altering Medications

Some hormonal agents alter the menstrual cycle and produce a "chemical menopause." Some of these are also used as treatment for endometriosis.

The results with PMS, as with other treatments, have not always been clear. These medications may have side effects similar to those of PMS. Taken over a long period of time, they can result in bone loss and other changes of menopause.

Diuretics

Diuretics (water pills) have been widely used for PMS, though they have had little success in alleviating most of the symptoms. While they do remove fluid from the body, they can also cause an increase in lethargy and dehydration. For women trying to lose weight, this fluid loss can result in confusion and unhappiness, since they often erroneously believe they have lost fat weight rather than water. The frequent combination of diuretic and laxative abuse results in women living in a constantly dehydrated and electrolyte-depleted state.

As we have discussed, simply drinking plain water may actually reduce bloating.

CHAPTER 16

❀

Alternative Therapies

Acupuncture

Eastern medicine views the mind and body as closely related and as made up of energy flows. Acupuncturists view PMS as an imbalance in the body's vital energy. Diagnosis involves determining whether the problem is one of excess energy, energy deficiency, or an energy blockage, and then knowing where, along the paths of energy flow, the imbalance is located. Fine needles are used to stimulate specific acupuncture points so that the flow of energy is regulated and blockages are removed. As with other treatments, it is not clear when acupuncture will or will not work. When successful, treatment may last for several months, with periodic "tune-ups" to maintain a balanced state.

As with all other treatments for PMS, there are practitioners and patients who claim that this is the one treatment that works. And for some it well may be. Women have sought acupuncture treatment before medical treatment, believing that it is more natural and safe. However, some have become worse before they have gotten better. Others have obtained relief immediately, and still others have gone on for many months with little improvement.

Currently some work is being done to investigate the biochemical effects of acupuncture. There is speculation that acupuncture affects neurotransmitter levels, which as described earlier have direct effects on the hypothalamus.

If you want to try acupuncture, it is important to find a qualified practitioner.

Chiropractic Adjustment

Many women have been relieved of their premenstrual symptoms after chiropractic treatments. Chiropractic is based on the principle that the entire body is affected by the spine; appropriate adjustment of the spine can therefore alleviate dysfunctional systems. This method is not well accepted within the medical community but has in fact offered considerable relief to many with PMS.

Other Methods

Acupressure, foot reflexology, therapeutic massage, and therapeutic touch are all systems of working with body energy to effect change. While they are only recently becoming widely used and accepted in Western medicine, these healing methods have been developed and used by other cultures for centuries. Although obviously you can apply pressure to your own foot or chest or other parts of the body, these techniques usually work best if someone else does them to/for you. In all healing there is the aspect of the healer and what that person brings to the method in terms of energy, desire to help, and technical skills.

The following methods of healing, as well as others that are similar, have at times been beneficial in reducing the immediate tension and stress of PMS. There are books about each of these techniques. Some of them are simple enough for you to learn with a partner so you can help each other. If you are going to use any of these methods, you must be prepared for the emotions that may be freed and expressed as a result of therapy. Working on the body often results in a surfacing of repressed feelings. Their expression may also be beneficial to you, but in any event, do not be surprised by their sometimes unexpected appearance.

ACUPRESSURE: Acupressure is similar to acupuncture but is conducted without needles. Pressure is applied to particular points on the body in order to change the flow of energy. Usually the points to be used are identified both by their location on body maps and by the pain produced when pressure is applied. However, even a light touch can give you some relief from symptoms.

FOOT REFLEXOLOGY: This unique method relies on identified points on the foot that correspond to both internal and external parts of the body. Special points are said to balance hormones. Foot reflexology can be relaxing and soothing for the entire body. Especially if you are somewhat anxious about having your body worked on, this is an extremely effective and nonthreatening way to introduce yourself to these methods. Foot reflexology requires removing only your socks or stockings. Results can feel quite similar to having had a total body massage.

THERAPEUTIC MASSAGE: Various forms of massage are designed to effect deeper changes in the body-tension level. Some are vigorous and others are quite gentle. Some can be done while you remain entirely clothed, while others require more direct access to your skin surface. Some of the gentler forms of massage allow for greater relaxation and deeper responses.

THERAPEUTIC TOUCH: This recently developed system, derived from ancient healing principles, is widely practiced by nurses and other health professionals. The practitioner works on the energy field around a person rather than directly on the body. It is done while you are fully clothed, simply sitting in a straight-backed chair. Energy is both felt and directed by the practitioner in order to give relief from symptoms.

Some of you may find these methods and even the language in which they are described to be quite strange. Others may be both surprised and relieved to see them described as healing modalities. PMS stretches us to grow. Its complexity, its pervasiveness, and its persistence often push us to search beyond culturally accepted procedures. For many women with PMS, treatment is a journey that motivates them to take risks in sharing their PMS experiences, in trying various kinds of treatment programs, and in looking for answers beyond those offered by traditional Western medicine.

CHAPTER 17

❁

Psychotherapy

Some women suffering from PMS have been helped and others hurt by traditional psychotherapy, depending on the views of the specific psychotherapist toward premenstrual tension and women's problems in general. Without a recognition of the biological component in premenstrual symptoms, the woman is made to feel that the changes she experiences are a result of psychopathology and that she ought to be able to prevent them. In fact, the *specific emotional* symptoms that a woman manifests premenstrually may be related to her particular personality, strengths, weaknesses, strivings, history, and drives. But the mood swings and the cyclic physiological changes are more a matter of her biological makeup.

Psychotherapy can be beneficial in helping a woman explore the specific emotional issues that upset her premenstrually. Whatever a woman is suppressing or trying to forget is likely to surface when she is premenstrual. Acknowledging and dealing with emotions usually bottled up or denied make them less likely to become overwhelming premenstrually.

Society discourages women from expressing anger, aggression, and ambition. The protective therapeutic relationship is often the beginning of a woman's ability to express anger and suppressed needs. Many women find it difficult to allow themselves comfort and pleasure. It often requires another person, a friend or a therapist, to help a woman begin to nurture and care for herself, to experience the self-love that is essential for well-being, to mother herself.

There are therefore real benefits to be gained from psychotherapy for the woman with PMS, providing the therapist and she recognize the full complexity of premenstrual changes and the interplay of body, mind, and emotion. The therapy must be directed at the integration of all these factors.

Keys to Successful Therapy

1. Find a qualified therapist who understands the interactions of body and mind, and who truly listens. Good therapists probably all begin with intuition and empathy, but they also require rigorous training and discipline. There are many avenues, however, to becoming a qualified therapist. Good ones may be psychologists, physicians, social workers, educators, pastoral counselors, et cetera, but they should have in common a prolonged, intensive, academic, and clinical education that prepares them to help others.

2. Have a commitment to facing hard questions, and be prepared to change. Change is never easy, or you wouldn't be seeking help.

3. Get referrals from friends who have been helped. Other sources are hospital or clinic referral services, or your other practitioners.

4. Interview, interview, interview. It may take consulting with more than one therapist before you choose someone to work with. It is perfectly acceptable to go for a consultation, or more than one, without making a commitment. You will learn something different from each person you see, and this will be useful knowledge as you proceed. Approach the choice as a good consumer would.

5. Set goals. Therapy should not be a lifetime activity. It should be organized so as to achieve specific aims over defined periods of time. It is important to set goals and time-frames, even though you may well change them. Reassess your progress periodically, alone and with your therapist.

6. A therapist should be chosen based on degree of skill, empathy, and intuition rather than the particular school or philosophy he or she represents. A study was once conducted in which tapes were made of several types of therapy sessions. The recorded dialogue from these sessions was almost indistinguishable in terms of philosophy or school. Therapy is about a competent and trusted person helping you.

CHAPTER 18

Support Groups

The object is to break the silence and to know that you are not alone.

Doctor, when you told me there had been other women whose PMS did not respond to any treatment, I suddenly didn't feel so alone anymore. I thought, there are others like me.

Consciousness-raising groups in the sixties and seventies helped many women validate their own experiences as women. Today, many hospitals, HMOs, and managed-care facilities offer support groups and networks for many of the health questions and problems of women.

The following are some guidelines for starting or finding such groups:

1. Look for ads or place an ad in a local paper, or try posting notices on bulletin boards at supermarkets, work (depending on how safe that feels), Y's, health clubs, or churches.

2. Set an initial time period—for instance, two or three months—to try a group, and then evaluate whether it is helpful.

3. If it is a leaderless group, rotate the leadership, with everyone taking a turn.

4. Remember that it's not just PMS problems that come to a group, but *women* with PMS as well as other social and medical problems that may or may not be related to the PMS. Don't try to cure everyone of everything.

5. Make a challenge of providing refreshments that are compatible with PMS dietary guidelines. (Don't forget popcorn!)

6. Create telephone trees for contacting people, both to create a support network and to ensure that the burden of the group does not fall on one or two people.

7. Rotate responsibilities regarding phone calls from/to new people seeking help or information.

8. Structure the group to allow each person to speak for a set time with no interruptions and to be sure every woman gets to talk before the discussion is thrown open to everyone.

9. Structure the time. If a meeting is to be three hours, allow time for "war stories" of suffering and past treatment difficulties and then go on to an agenda. This allows people a chance both to vent feelings and then to be involved in some constructive planning and support. Use the contents page of this or any other book about PMS as a guideline for each week.

10. You may want to learn some alternative healing methods together so you can help one another during difficult times. For instance, some or all of you can attend massage or foot-reflexology workshops, or you may be able to have a practitioner give a workshop for the whole group.

11. Try role-playing of premenstrual personalities. This is difficult at first, but as you begin to share your "monsters," they lose some of their frightening and controlling aspects.

12. Don't forget humor. In the worst of it all, the ability to laugh at oneself can be lifesaving.

Support groups can occasionally generate stress or trauma. Some PMS groups have ended with disappointment or bitterness. While this can happen with any group, there are some particular problems and pitfalls for women starting and belonging to PMS groups:

· Coming to define one's life by PMS. There is more to life than PMS, but it is easy, especially when you are experiencing the enthusiasm of validation, for life to become centered around PMS.

· Burnout from trying to take care of all the needs of others. Learning to help and also to say no is always a challenge.

· The belief that one's own PMS has to be cured before one can be helpful to others. The persistence of PMS symptoms has to be understood by everyone because the group will have to deal with all the tensions and mood swings characteristics of PMS. It doesn't necessarily go away because you are a leader or a member of a PMS group.

· Anger over disruptive behavior of a group member who is having PMS. In a way, the PMS group gives women a chance to experience what those around them experience on a regular basis when they are suffering from PMS.

· Competition over whose PMS is worst and who has the worst horror stories.

Support groups will not cure PMS, but they can make it more manageable. One of the most devastating aspects of any illness is the isolation it can create. There is no way to underestimate how important it is to be in a group with others "like me." People move, having to leave familiar places, friends, and family. Groups, by definition, counteract isolation.

PART III

Broader Aspects of PMS

CHAPTER 19

❀

Sexuality
and PMS

Talk is to girls as sex is to boys.

Margaret lay in bed staring at the ceiling. Restless, she tried not to move, aware of Jake on the other side of the bed. They lay facing away from each other, the strain of their fighting showing in the distance between them. She knew he'd be asleep soon and the long night would be hers alone, and silent.

Maybe, if her sleep were quiet, she too would be able to rest. But instead she had nightmares in which she kept losing control. A part of her wished she could lean over and touch Jake's body, feel the warmth that at times made all her other fears disappear. What if she did move closer? What was the price of reaching across? She wasn't proud of the words she had spoken. Would the anger she expressed to him come back at her? She knew her last spate of accusations had hit him deeply. She listened to his breathing, guessing that he was still awake but that he wanted her to believe he was asleep. It was another piece of his withdrawal. If she moved over, if she touched him, would he also think she was taking back everything she had said? Would he think she wanted to make love, when what she craved was tender words?

"Self-contained," that's how she usually thought of herself, but tonight the restlessness in her body made her want to fling herself away from her confusion, her unexpected fears, anger, tears. "I'm self-contained and self-sufficient," she thought, "except lately I haven't been that way very much."

Sometimes she imagined that her anger at Jake came from knowing she could not reach across to ask him to hold her. Before she could even express her needs to him, she was angry for his presumed refusal. And what if he thought she wanted to make love? How could she tell him she wanted only to be held? Sex is a mystery, and years of marriage, books, and talking had not made it any clearer. Recently she hadn't wanted to make love a lot of the time, and that had put its own strain on their relationship. Doing it when she didn't want to was terrible. Tonight she wanted to be held and didn't want sex. Jake usually had trouble with that. He'd get angry, and then they'd be fighting again.

Margaret doesn't have to have PMS to be in her current situation. In fact, hers is not an uncommon experience for women in our culture. The issues raised here regarding sexuality are relevant to women with PMS and without it. However, the importance of PMS to sexuality is that most women with PMS do experience some change in their sex drive premenstrually. Some have a greatly increased sex drive, while others lose theirs altogether. Depression is usually associated with a decreased libido, but in PMS there is not always a clear association. A woman can be premenstrually depressed and withdrawn and still have an increased sex drive, although the opposite—a decreased drive—is more common.

Premenstrually some women also find that their body changes in ways affecting their sexuality. Breast tenderness can be so severe as to make any touching of the nipples painful, while at the same time sexual feelings can be strong and compelling. Bloating can make a woman feel both uncomfortable and unattractive.

Body size is often as much a matter of fashion as of health. There is a story told of an anthropologist visiting an African tribe and seeing a young woman dramatically tugging hard at her firm breasts. When queried, she explained that she was trying to make them hang the way a grown woman's are supposed to, which in that culture was a sign of maturity. Without our own cultural bias toward thinness, premenstrual women might even be able to boast about their cyclically protruding abdomens. Women, of course, say that they feel better when they are not bloated, but some of that sense of well-being comes from seeing ourselves through other people's eyes. Nothing kills libido or self-esteem quite like feeling ugly.

Sensuality, the need to touch and be touched, to hold and be held, must be differentiated from genital sexuality. Many women have an increased need for intimacy premenstrually while at the same time being either neutral or repelled by sexuality. This can be confusing to the woman as well as to her partner, who may interpret the overtures toward intimacy as initiating sex.

Sexuality cannot be separated from the people engaged in a sexual or potentially sexual relationship. All the dynamics of PMS, which play themselves out in other areas, will also exist within the realm of sexuality. How a woman feels about herself and her sexuality will play a part in how her premenstrual sexual changes are expressed. A woman who is in a celibate relationship will experience a premenstrually increased libido differently from a woman who is sexually active in a relationship. The change in her drive will have different meanings and consequences for both her and her partner.

For instance, a woman with an increased sex drive premenstrually can seek out her partner and express her sexual needs. She can seek out new partners. She can masturbate. She can remain sexually stimulated and take no action toward having those needs met. Which option a woman chooses will depend on how she feels about herself, her sexuality, whether she is in a primary relationship, how she feels about touching herself and masturbating, and so forth. And at different times in her life she may choose differently.

For women with decreased libido, the issues are slightly different and more often depend on what is happening in an ongoing sexual relationship. For instance:

- To what extent does she feel she has a choice about how and when she has sexual relations?
- Is her premenstrual lack of desire specific to one person?
- Is her desire marginal anyway and simply absent premenstrually?
- Is she free to express her needs for affection without sexuality, and is her partner receptive to those needs?
- Is the lack of sexual desire connected to an increase in psychological vulnerability?

• Are there sexual conflicts when she's not premenstrual?
• Can she separate issues of premenstrual irritability, anxiety, anger, or depression from sexual needs?

A Sexual Inventory

Looking at your own views about sexuality can be helpful in understanding and coping with premenstrual sexual changes. The following questions are meant to stimulate thought on the subject. They do not have right or wrong answers but are intended to help simplify what is often experienced as an entanglement of sexuality.

1. What are your basic beliefs about sexuality?

2. What are your feelings about touching yourself, sexual play, masturbation, or making love to yourself? It is amazing how many women have read or heard enough to believe that it is normal for children to masturbate but have not been able to believe that this is also true for themselves.

3. Have most of your sexual experiences been gratifying for you? Have you experienced orgasm? With a partner? By yourself? Spontaneously?

4. Have you ever found yourself using sex as a favor or withholding it as a punishment?

5. What are your feelings about initiating sexual activity?

6. Do you feel you can refuse to have sex?

7. What are your religious beliefs about sex?

8. Are you afraid of your partner?

9. Is your partner afraid of you?

10. The assumption is that we are all modern and liberated these days, but what are your feelings about sex in relation to sin, shame, guilt, pleasure, and punishment?

11. Do you feel free to talk about sexuality with your partner or partners when you have them? (An anomaly of our culture is that many people will

easily take off their clothes and have sex with someone else but will not feel free to talk with that person about it.)

12. Do you feel free to express what you like/dislike in sexuality?

13. Do you feel your partner has the right to say no? Do you get angry? Do you feel hurt?

14. How are your feelings about sexuality related to your feelings about your body? For example, do you think of your sexuality as being related to your weight or fitness?

Take some time to look over this questionnaire. Many of these questions may take a long time to answer, and you may have different answers for them at different times in your life. Keep in mind both your general answers and how they may vary during the menstrual cycle. For example, you may feel comfortable about initiating sexual activity, but premenstrually you may *need* your partner to take more initiative. Or you may think of yourself as someone who enjoys her sexuality, but premenstrually you just don't want to be touched at all.

Sexuality and PMS Treatment

Treatment for PMS may or may not affect sexual aspects of the cyclic changes. Obviously, if women are less depressed, less angry, and less anxious, their sexual responses will be more directly connected to their feelings about sexuality and their relationships. As couples begin to develop ways of communicating about PMS and sexuality changes, they also will be able to be more responsive to each other. Compromise and communication by both partners can lead to more satisfying relationships.

One of the more common dynamics of a couple is for the woman with PMS to withdraw sexually when she is premenstrual and for her partner to be threatened by this withdrawal and to want sexual relations even more. Often the more one person pulls away, the more the other is in pursuit. Even if a couple is having sexual relations once a week, for example, the withdrawal may leave the other partner wanting it daily, as reassurance that the relationship and its sexual component are intact. Treatment of PMS along with explanations of dynamics such as these often help a couple to get through the premenstrual period with their relationship intact, even if there is no actual change in the frequency of sexual contact.

Problems of decreased libido have to date been the PMS symptoms least responsive to therapy, and this holds true even for medical treatments. Progesterone for some women causes a decrease in sexual drive even if there wasn't a pronounced cyclic depression in that drive previously.

Problems of increased sex drive have been somewhat easier to deal with, since these tend to be less threatening to most relationships. The changes in sexuality associated with PMS are not a problem per se unless the woman and her partner view them as such.

CHAPTER 20

❁

The Family
and PMS

He asked how he could help, and I said, "Love me through it."

PMS affects women, and when women are part of a family, it affects the family. When a mother has PMS, when a teenage daughter has PMS, when a grandmother has PMS, the entire family group may feel it.

Women differ as to who receives the brunt of their PMS. Some women turn it inward and become depressed or suicidal; others turn on partners, children, or colleagues. The inconsistency and unpredictability of mood swings are usually the most difficult aspects of PMS for the woman and others. Remember, however, everyone has moods, needs, problems, anger, and conflicts in relationships.

While there are some women whose PMS simply goes away with treatment, many other women and their families must continue to grapple with some cyclic mood swings. In certain families there may be a residue of emotions that continue to affect everyone even after the PMS itself is under control. And in still others, the PMS was never really the major problem, and its resolution has made more obvious the ways in which the family is struggling.

Husbands and PMS

Men do not get PMS, but when they are close to a woman with PMS, they become involved in the dynamics of the problems. Men don't make PMS happen, but at times their own personality traits contribute to the premenstrual discord. In our society, women tend to be more emotional, or at least more expressive of the emotions they have, and are even more openly emotional premenstrually. Thus a relationship already strained by a discrepancy in expressiveness will be even more strained when the woman is premenstrual. Most of the women I have talked to, both with and without PMS, have described their husbands or boyfriends as rarely talking about personal problems, not being emotional, "keeping everything in," and often being angry at the woman's need for expression.

Silas, in the following anecdote, is like many men I have seen with their wives, men who have come to talk about their wives or lovers, and men who have been described to me by unhappy and, at times, lonely women. In comparison with most of these men, he is neither the most macho nor the most sensitive. And like most of them, Silas is indeed trying his best.

Silas slouched in the crushed-velvet armchair of the doctor's office and stared silently at the slightly off-center portrait on the far wall. Therapy was a concession to his wife and their marriage counselor. He didn't want to be here, but he was willing to give it a try. He wanted to make their lives together better, but this office, the words spoken here, were foreign to him.

"Women are the emotional center of the family." That's what had been said several sessions before, and Silas had no disagreement with that statement. Mothers were emotional. His mother had been, his wife was. His father hadn't been, and neither was he. In spite of all the recent propaganda telling boys it was okay to cry, Silas found a certain comfort in the old order, in a clarity that defined men's and women's needs and their expressions differently. Why change it? Why change anything?

Sure, sometimes life had its pains, but you kept a stiff upper lip and went on.

But each month, before Elizabeth, his wife, got her period, the lid was loosened off a cauldron of resentments. She'd say something cutting, and suddenly Silas's face would flush, his arms and chest would become tight, and he'd have to sit very still so that he wouldn't explode. Even as he thought about it, he could feel his body tensing. Her emotions frightened him.

Listening to the therapist, Silas was reluctant to engage in the difficult task of communicating. He remembered being three years old and seeing words on a page. At the time he couldn't imagine how those symbols would ever make sense to him. Once he'd learned to read, though, it was odd remembering not being able to read. He wondered if that would ever be true for this experience.

He forced his attention back to the room, to the therapist, and to what he was supposed to be doing here. He was supposed to talk, and then somehow their marriage was supposed to get better. Still, there was something good about getting it off his chest, even if it didn't change anything. Women expressed their feelings, and men got it off their chests.

"I can't seem to make her happy," Silas said. "At that time of the month, everything I do is wrong."

Silas's wife has PMS, and they as a couple have difficulties. Even without PMS, there are times when they are in conflict. Silas feels confused, as if something is being asked of him that he can't understand. Elizabeth feels isolated because he can't seem to hear what she is saying or be sympathetic or supportive.

The belief that all will be well when a woman's PMS is treated is a fantasy that assigns all the family's troubles to the woman and her PMS. Unfortunately, treatment may not only leave areas of conflict unresolved but may even accentuate other problems in the relationship.

> *He hits me when I'm premenstrual. I know I provoke him,*
> *but every time it happens, I'm still surprised. I feel so bad*
> *about myself, I think I must have deserved this. Then, after*
> *my period, I get angry with myself for letting him do that to*
> *me and for staying with him.*

Sometimes the woman with PMS seems to express emotions for both herself and her partner. Although dreaded, the explosions become an emotional purge for everyone involved. In a marriage, the woman's anger often becomes an excuse for the man to let go of his. When the woman gains more control over her emotions and this dynamic changes, the couple is left without this outlet and must begin to develop new ways of releasing tension, both individually and/or together.

When I have PMS, we all have PMS.

In a family with identified PMS, the mother often takes on the responsibility for everyone's moods. When she isn't cool, calm, or collected, she is considered ill, while others may act out anger, irritability, and even violence in "response" to her illness.

On the other hand, women with PMS often have an uncanny ability to lash out at another person's most vulnerable areas. They can be most insensitive and destructive, often deeply regretting what they have said but nonetheless leaving the other person devastated and confused.

PMS is not confined to women in heterosexual relationships. Lesbian women seeking treatment for PMS and their partners often describe their difficulties with the relationship in words identical to women with PMS and their male partners. The same premenstrual tensions, accusations, and withdrawal exist. When the couple's menstrual cycles become synchronous and therefore both women are premenstrual at approximately the same time, the tensions, strains, and potential for explosions are even greater. Women tend to believe that they are more understanding than men of other women's suffering, but they can be as frustrated, impatient, needy, and vulnerable as the male partners of women with PMS.

PMS has at times been used by women as an excuse for abuse. People in relationships cannot be expected to suffer abuse just because the behavior has a medical name. Painful things are said and done. Though you may be sympathetic to a woman's PMS, there is still a need to get some distance, to protect yourself from the behavioral effects of PMS, whether these are physical or emotional. Separation can, at times, be helpful.

Teens, Moods, and PMS

Adolescence in our culture is a serious challenge—for the girl or boy, and for families, schools, and the community. Moodiness and lack of predictability are the norm at this time.

PMS can start with menarche, the time of a girl's first menstrual period. To differentiate the general mood swings of adolescence from premenstrual changes is difficult, if not impossible. Teenagers tend to be much less articulate than adults about how they are feeling. They tend to deny any connection between their moods and their cycles. The association may imply that the moods are less real or that their feelings are less valid.

Carly's diary illustrates some of these conflicts:

Thursday night

Dear Diary,

You must think that all I ever feel is sad because that's when I write to you. That's not true, though. Sometimes I feel really happy, but I guess I only need to write to you when I'm unhappy.

Today I'm unhappy and yesterday I was unhappy. Sometimes there is a good reason, but other times I just feel unhappy and then I find reasons. Like if someone says something to me one day it can be okay, but on another day I get angry at them or angry at myself.

My face . . . Sometimes I think I'm ugly, that my hair is ugly, that I'm fat, my legs are too fat. A voice inside me just whines with all the things wrong with me.

At school today I was standing in the lunch line and I saw Evie and Tori having lunch together and I just felt left out. Suddenly my eyes got red and I thought I was going to cry right there. I got out a tissue and pretended I had to sneeze, and then I started coughing so my red eyes wouldn't show so much. This is stupid. Why should I care? They're both creeps anyway. Then I came home and started working on the report due in history and I couldn't concentrate. It's stupid anyway. Who cares about kings? Kings are creeps.

Today in English class I couldn't concentrate at all. I kept thinking about a poem I wanted to write. The teacher got mad at me because she saw me writing notes, and when she called on me I was off in space and couldn't remember which book we were supposed to be reading. She said she is calling my mother because I keep doing this . . . something about not living up to my potential, I think.

Next month I'll be fifteen. If I live to seventy-five that's one fifth of my lifetime gone already. I might not even live that long.

Tuesday afternoon

Dear Diary,

Last night I pigged out on two Reese's marshmallow fudge sundaes and a bag of chocolate chip cookies. This morning my face looks horrible and I HATE myself and I HATE everyone else too.

I yelled at Evie in the locker room because her bag pushed my towel onto the floor. YUK... I told her I didn't ever want to be her friend again. The locker room is filthy. I hate getting undressed and then dressed again to go to stupid dances.

Thank God I can shut the door to this room and be alone. If anyone else says anything to me I'll hit them. Why is it some days everything goes wrong?

Carly's mother would not do well to say, "Carly, maybe you are premenstrual."

Carly may or may not have PMS. She does have moods, as do most adolescents, female and male. Only by charting can we relate her moods to her menstrual period. And if they are related, there is still the question as to whether we should consider anything to be wrong with her. If her moods are troublesome to her, she may want to try altering her diet, exercising, et cetera. If her moods are troublesome only for her family, she still has to decide if she wants to try to change herself at all. It does not work for the family to try to change an adolescent's PMS, just as it does not work for a spouse to try to treat a woman's PMS.

An important exception is with women who are retarded or mentally incompetent and unable to take care of themselves. In that event, support people may begin treatment regimens to try to affect disturbing cyclic behavior by using diet changes or medications. In general it just doesn't work to try to treat someone else's PMS. Even with medication, there needs to be active cooperation on the part of the woman with PMS in order to achieve any success.

Telling Children About PMS

One day I cleaned out my daughter's closet, locked myself inside, and screamed into a pillow. Later my son asked me if I'd heard a strange sound in the house.

Babies, toddlers, and young children are confused by mood changes. As they get older, children are better able to understand the inconsistencies of a mother suffering from PMS. Eventually they are even able to consciously modify their own behavior in relation to a mother's needs at some times of the month.

> *Pretend that sometimes Mommy is inside a balloon and she needs some quiet and needs for you all to be gentle with her.*

> *Some days of the month Mommy yells when chores aren't done, and other days she just laughs and tells you to do them. Can you figure out which days those are, and would you like to write them down?*

However, children have their own needs, including the need for emotional release. They often know when a request will bring a yes and when it will provoke irritation or anger. When irritable or moody themselves, they can be adept at both inciting adult explosions and becoming the target of those explosions.

> *Eventually the boys learned that there were certain times when I needed to be left alone. Sometimes it was just to take a bath without being interrupted.*

Living in a culture in which we try to give our children the best, we find it hard to come to terms with our own shortcomings as parents. Guilt becomes a major obstacle to sharing the facts about PMS with our children. We don't want our children to have a "sick" parent. When the illness is barely understood and the reality of it is often doubted, the problems are confounded. Children can become caught in marital conflict over PMS, and most often this is conflict reflecting and expressing their father's anger toward their mother.

Can women with PMS be good mothers? Of course they can, depending on the severity of their problems and their ability to deal with them. As repeatedly stated, PMS can be mild or severe. It can interfere in some areas of a woman's life and not in others. And it is treatable.

Both mothers and fathers have moods. Although one question might be "Is Mommy premenstrual?" another should be "What mood will Daddy be in when he comes home tonight?" Men and women get angry.

Feelings of anger and actions are not the same and should not be confused.

Points to Remember for Women with PMS and Their Families

1. PMS affects the entire family.

2. All family members have moods.

3. Identifying PMS does not make all the problems go away.

4. Treatment of PMS may not make all the problems go away.

5. Family support is important in lifestyle and dietary changes.

6. Some family problems may be related to PMS, and others may not.

7. Family members can be both victims and instigators of premenstrual explosions.

8. Being premenstrual is not an illness. Having moods is not an illness. Having severe premenstrual symptoms that interfere with your life is an illness.

9. The woman with PMS must be responsible for her treatment. Others can only support her.

CHAPTER 21

❖

Creativity
and PMS

I feel receptive premenstrually, and more sensitive. I take everything in, but I can't discriminate well. Then later I have to try to figure it all out.

I get scared I'll get lost in my work. I'm in a frenzy with it, and then I get my period and I'm different again.

I get surges of energy premenstrually and suddenly want to clean, move furniture, or write. These are real highs and lows.

For me sexual energy and creative energy seem to come at the same time in my cycle. For a while I'm driven crazy by both, but I get a lot done and then I menstruate and I feel normal again.

Women may have a lessening of boundaries, of control, and of rules during the premenstrual time. They seem to be directed more by what is occurring internally than externally. While this can obviously lead to difficulties in living, it can also stimulate creative expression. Along with the lessening of constraint, there is also a heightened sensitivity to sound, sight, and smell. Colors may take on a different hue.

While creativity may be enhanced premenstrually, putting expression into form may be a challenge. An artist may find her creative ideas and colors premenstrually but do her best finished work *after* she gets her period.

One artist said:

> *I do sketches when I am premenstrual. That's when I get*
> *my ideas, but I never start the full drawing then. I can't get*
> *the lines the way I want them. I see them, but I can't do it*
> *right on the paper.*

Defining or explaining creativity may not be any easier than explaining God. We watch as children create on the beach making sand castles. Musicians create by playing their instruments. Women create by knitting or crocheting. Artists are creative in their painting or sculpting. They are all drawing on inner images of how something is to take shape. In each case, the final form reflects both agreed-upon societal patterns as well as an individual imprint.

What we usually do not consider creative is replicating what has been done—tracing a drawing, constructing a building exactly the same as all the others, turning over a pail of sand and saying that it's a castle. So creativity includes some individuality and some variation from standard blueprints. Premenstrually, many women are more aware of inner visions and less attached to blueprints.

Creativity has been tied to suffering. Whether in fact this is true, it does appear that some people can use their pain creatively. To the extent that PMS alters consciousness and produces pain, it can at times be a catalyst for new growth and meaning.

> *I would never have wished for PMS, but as a result of my*
> *illness I have a new and deeper understanding of others' suf-*
> *fering. I'd had an easy life until PMS. I hope now to help*
> *others who are in pain.*

CHAPTER 22

❊

Social and Political Implications

MEDICAL TRENDS, LIKE MANY THINGS, occur within a political context. They grow out of the presumptions and ethics of a particular time. The apparent "rediscovery" in 1981 of an old problem coincided with a renewed campaign for women's equality. Recognition of PMS emerged as the Equal Rights Amendment was being defeated. The relationship between premenstrual tension and hormones had already been described in 1931 by Dr. Robert T. Frank. Dr. Katharina Dalton had been talking and writing about PMS since 1953. Then for years it was ignored, and women who did suffer were given inappropriate advice and made to feel at times that they were imagining the problem.

PMS "arrived" in the United States on the heels of British court cases in which women pleaded that their violent actions were the result of their uncontrollable PMS; this caught the attention of millions of women who finally felt validated in their own experiences of cyclic physical and emotional disturbances. At the same time, it created some conflict within groups struggling for equal opportunities for women. Many feared that the recognition of PMS would result in a political setback for women, who would be portrayed, once again, as undependable, out of control, flawed, and therefore unworthy of political office, well-paying jobs, or custody of their own children.

Few women, however, actually lose control premenstrually. A woman with severe PMS will be limited by her symptoms. One with mild mood changes will not. In the same way, a man with an illness may or may not be limited by that illness. This issue is not about *all* women.

The particular mood expressions of PMS must also be seen in the context of a society that discourages women's anger, ambition, and independence. Sometimes this discouragement is overt, and other times it is a matter of voices that have been internalized by the woman herself. The husband of a woman who came for help described their problem as follows:

> *My wife is fine for two weeks out of the month. She's friendly and a good wife. The house is clean. Then she ovulates, and suddenly she's not happy about her life. She wants a job. She wants to go back to school. Then her period comes, and she is all right again.*

One woman said:

> *I'm a happy person with a good life. I have a husband who is good to me and three healthy children. Then when I'm premenstrual these thoughts come into my head like "What is the meaning of my life?" I don't have room for those thoughts! I just want them to go away.*

PMS and Responsibility

The issue of responsibility and PMS is a confusing one: "Is it my PMS or is it me?"

Each woman experiences PMS somewhat differently, has more or less anger or sadness or irritability. If one woman expresses her PMS as suicidal fantasy and another as homicidal, then these two women have in their personalities certain destructive energies directed either toward themselves or toward others. There is no evidence for one kind of PMS that makes a woman suicidal as opposed to another that makes her homicidal, or creative, or causes her to shoplift. PMS is the feeling, not the expression.

I first learned of hypnosis as a child. My friends and I would talk about this mysterious force that would make you do something you would never do on your own. Then as I grew older I learned that hypnosis could not make you be or do something that was totally against who you were and what your values were. I am still not sure what the real truth is about that, but the situation is similar in PMS. For the most part, people do not do things contrary to their values, even when they are suffering from PMS.

The antisocial behavior of PMS is probably more a matter of premenstrual magnification (PMM) than of PMS. The women in England who committed crimes had histories of prior and subsequent antisocial behavior. To say that the premenstrual state magnified these impulses is more correct than to say that PMS caused their behavior.

PMS does seem to lessen the control with which people restrain impulses, and it seems to lessen their ability to deal with disturbing inner images. But the particular means of expression seems distinctly individual. No one's Mr. Hyde is exactly like another's. We all have had nightmares or bad dreams. My nightmares and yours may have similar themes, but there are individual differences specific to who I am and who you are. If my dreams or fantasies begin to seep into waking reality and I begin to act as if they are real, is that me? The weakening of boundaries may be biological, emotional, or spiritual. At what point am I considered to have lost control? When am I responsible for what I have done as a result of having those dreams come into reality? These questions have no clear answers.

The questions become even more confusing when they relate to law. Law is a system of dealing with rules for a society and may not have much to do with truth, morality, or biology. The courts may decide issues concerning PMS and women's responsibility for their actions, but they don't answer the question of whether women are or are not responsible. They will say only how the legal system decides to view PMS, and other human disorders, at a certain point in history.

Legally defining women as not responsible will add to undesirable stereotypes of women. This defense, as any, may also be exploited by women who are unwilling to take responsibility for their actions, in the same way that men and women can exploit similar laws governing sanity and responsibility.

The issue is emotionally charged. Like abortion, it combines aspects of personal behavior and beliefs with societal rules and definition. Both men and women have very strong feelings about PMS, and arguments are often based on those emotions. Court decisions will have little impact on such emotions.

Ultimately, we have no uniform way of deciding responsibility at any one time for any person. If six psychiatrists are trying to determine whether someone is responsible for a crime, some will see it one way and some another. And even if six people agree, whether they be six psychiatrists or six people off the street, that only means that they agree, not that they have determined the truth.

The question of responsibility is broader than PMS but is nevertheless relevant. If we see ourselves as products of unfortunate circumstances or bodily processes, does that relieve us of responsibility for our actions? If a person is abused as a child, is that person not responsible for his or her actions in abusing children as an adult? To hold someone responsible does not negate the circumstances that may have contributed to those actions; to not hold someone responsible may do a disservice to those who have survived past or present hardships and have been able, often through great pain and struggle, to overcome destructive patterns of behavior.

The Other Side of PMS

Many years ago I tried thinking about PMS in its reverse form. In other words, what if we looked at the other side of PMS, or that time of month when a woman is *not* premenstrual?

If a woman has PMS, what is she like when she is not premenstrual? If she is overly emotional premenstrually, is she overly repressed the rest of the month? Which is real? Which is she? Does the answer have to be that one is real and the other isn't? She may well be both, but one is more socially acceptable.

The list of characteristics I describe below evolved from years of listening to women's stories. These women's menstrual cycles were a source of difficulty, but so were the demands put on them by others, and even more, demands that they put on themselves. The "symptoms" on the next page occur "around" the follicular phase.

PERIFOLLICULAR REPRESSIVE SYNDROME: THE OTHER SIDE OF PMS

A condition characterized by the following symptoms that begin within a few days of menstruation and end at ovulation:

1. Presence of a fixed belief, often of delusional proportion, that one is sprung from the extra rib of Clark Kent, thus believing oneself to be superwoman.
2. Lack of anger in the presence of a husband or partner who is inattentive, absent, or overly demanding.
3. Inability to become irritated when in the company of three or more children over the course of twelve to sixteen hours.
4. Inability to maintain sufficient fluid levels in abdominal and breast tissue, so that clothing that fits correctly in the premenstrual phase hangs loosely during the follicular phase.
5. Inability to take a day off from work when feeling ill.
6. Lack of interest in chocolate or salty foods.
7. Fixed belief regarding the necessity of a clean and orderly house in the presence of rain, snow, mud, children, spouse, pets, and company.
8. Inability to weep at sad events.
9. Extreme guilt regarding inability to maintain standards of perfection.

"Who am I?" does not have a static answer. We are dynamic, not isolated from our bodies or our environments. That is our human quality, irrespective of gender.

APPENDIX

❀

Getting Help
for PMS

PMS IS PERSISTENT, AND EVEN with self-help solutions, it may not go away or it may recur if it *has* gone away. At various times, you may want to seek medical care for your PMS because you:

- need confirmation that you have PMS.
- have symptoms that are interfering with your sense of well-being.
- have symptoms that interfere with your functioning.
- find that self-help hasn't been enough.
- feel that self-help may be more than you can manage.

Finding adequate medical care for this condition can be difficult depending on the availability of knowledgeable practitioners, health insurance, and your financial resources.

Some physicians still resist recognizing and treating PMS, a tendency that is not necessarily dependent on the gender of the physician. Female and male doctors may be equally insensitive to PMS. Women need to consider these factors as they seek and assess medical care for their PMS.

In no health situation should you simply approach your physician or other health care provider and say, "Fix me." That is especially true in PMS, where the consumer may know more about the subject than the doctor and where many of the treatments are experimental and may require extreme lifestyle changes.

In any health situation, your own attitudes partly influence how you are treated. This is tricky in PMS, where many women come to a physician with vulnerability about being believed, with gratitude for any attention or help, but also with many resentments about past experiences seeking help.

Asking your medical practitioner the following questions may be helpful in approaching medical care for PMS.

1. What causes PMS? (The answer to this will tell you much about this professional's knowledge and attitudes about both PMS and women's problems.)

2. What are the possible therapies for PMS? (Look for breadth of answers.)

3. Which ones has this practitioner used and why?

4. What is this practitioner's favorite, or the one with which he/she is most successful?

5. What are the risks of each treatment?

6. What are the costs of each treatment?

Coming to terms with PMS often involves going through stages of anger, acceptance, blaming all your troubles on PMS, a sense of betrayal by your own body, resentment of previous practitioners, and unrealistic expectations. All of these are normal reactions to the discovery of PMS or validation of longtime difficulties. Recognition of their presence may make obtaining future help easier and more fruitful.

As you search for help with your PMS, take your charts with you and believe in your own story. Look to professionals for their skills and guidance but not necessarily for validation of your own truths.

In every person there is a drive toward health. Some healing can be accomplished on your own, some with the help of others, both friends and professionals. A sense of self-empowerment is the foundation for seeking and receiving help in the treatment of phenomena related to the menstrual cycle.

Using the Internet

There is an abundance of women's health information on the Internet. If you haven't yet used the Internet or aren't sure if you want to, your local library is the best place to explore this possibility. Many libraries now have computers where community members can get onto the Internet, and some even offer courses on how to use this powerful tool.

The Internet can seem intimidating to the uninitiated, but once you understand a few very simple concepts you'll feel more comfortable about using it. Simply defined, the Internet is a network of computer files linked together. These files may contain text, graphics, or even animation and music. On the Internet, you can look at these files on your computer screen and follow the "web" of links to similar or related files.

How does it work? A *browser* (for example, Netscape, Internet Explorer) is a type of computer program that allows you to see files on the Internet. Once your browser gives you access to the Internet, you use a *search engine* (for example Excite, Yahoo!) to scan the Internet and display the files you want to see. For instance, if you point your mouse to "search" and type in "PMS," your search engine will display the names of literally thousands of files on PMS. To narrow the number of files, focus your search in a specific area, for example, "herbal remedies for PMS" or "serotonin levels and PMS."

For women with PMS, the Internet can be useful to:

- locate medical-journal and other articles about PMS.
- read about PMS remedies, including prescription and nonprescription treatments.
- identify medical facilities where PMS is treated or where research is being conducted.
- connect with other women who have PMS.

In some ways, the benefits of using the Internet to retrieve information and connect with other women and health organizations are the same as the disadvantages associated with this tool:

- **The amount of information.** Since entering *PMS* will retrieve literally thousands of files, it takes patience and skill to sort out the information and to distinguish between credible information and unfounded claims designed to sell products.

· The ability of information to be dispersed rapidly. Connecting with others who have similar health issues can be powerful. Do safeguard your privacy, and be cautious about giving out information on the Internet. Verify all you can about any organization you contact via the Internet— where it is, how long it has existed, what products or services are available. When communicating with other people on the Internet, either in chat rooms, news groups, or through E-mail messages, think carefully about revealing your address, phone number, or other personal information.

The Internet will not help you find an individual approach to managing PMS that will work for you. However, the information and support available there may become valuable components of the self-care program you design to meet your needs.

Recognizing PMS and finding ways to take care of it is ultimately a journey of self-discovery and self-empowerment. The tools or methods you use will vary widely, but in the end you will be able to overcome the obstacles that PMS presents to you. There will be a time when you can look back and say, "Gee, PMS? I used to have that trouble!"

In the earliest years of PMS in the United States, many of us believed that PMS support groups would flourish and become a permanent part of the women's health care landscape. In the beginning there were many such groups, partly because information was so difficult to find. But once women got their PMS under control or eliminated it altogether, many of them simply wanted to get on with their lives. The "sickness" model was replaced by one of health. Vulnerability was replaced by strength.

Listed below are books and other resources for help with PMS. They are the tools for understanding and treating PMS, for making your journey from vulnerability to strength.

Books

Bender, Stephanie. *Women Tell Women How to Control Premenstrual Syndrome.* Oakland, CA: New Harbinger Publications, 1996.
A helpful guide that discusses the effects of PMS on self-esteem, relationships, family, and work.

Bennet, William, and Joel Gurin. *The Dieter's Dilemma.* New York: Basic Books, 1982.

Useful to women with PMS trying to lose weight without fasting or stringent dieting. Excellent discussion of body size.

Birch, Beryl Bender. *Power Yoga: The Total Strength and Flexibility Workout.* New York: Fireside, 1995.
Good resource for beginners interested in yoga for strength and relaxation.

Boston Women's Health Book Collective. *The New Our Bodies, Ourselves.* New York: Touchstone Books, 1996.
A classic in women's health, now expanded and updated. Essential reading for any woman wanting to learn more about her body.

Capacchione, Lucia. *The Creative Journal.* Athens, OH: New Castle, 1988.
An excellent collection of journal exercises that use writing and drawing for self-awareness.

Carrington, Patricia. *Freedom in Meditation,* Second Edition. Kendall Park, NJ: Pace Educational Systems, 1984.
Comprehensive discussion of meditation, its history and current uses. Detailed instruction and guidelines on how to meditate.

————. *Releasing.* New York: William Morrow, 1984.
An excellent guide to letting go of self-defeating involvement with particular people or problems in your life. Step-by-step instructions to relieve stress and tension.

Christensen, Alice. *20-Minute Yoga Workouts.* New York: Fawcett, 1995.
Quick exercises; particularly helpful if you want to alternate yoga with other forms of exercise.

Copeland, Mary Ellen. *The Depression Workbook.* Oakland, CA: New Harbinger Publications, 1992.
Insightful exercises to help manage mood swings and depression.

Dalton, Katharina. *Once a Month.* Alameda, CA: Hunter House, 1997.
Dr. Dalton's classic work on PMS, now in its fifth edition, broke the silence on this disorder. Dr. Dalton sees women purely as victims of their bodies and men as victims of their women. Progesterone is described as the single solution to PMS.

————. *The Premenstrual Syndrome and Progesterone Therapy.* Chicago: Year Book Medical Pubs., 1977.
For medical practitioners, a discussion of progesterone and a guide to its use.

Dan, Alice J., Effie A. Graham, and Carol P. Beecher, eds. *The Menstrual Cycle,* Volume 1. New York: Springer, 1980.
A valuable collection of papers by scholars in different disciplines. Often critical of previous research and theory about the menstrual cycle.

Debrovner, C., ed. *Premenstrual Tension.* New York: Human Sciences Press, 1982.
Written for professionals, this book contains various approaches to PMS treatment.

Edwards, Betty. *Drawing on the Right Side of the Brain.* Los Angeles: J. P. Tarcher, 1989.
This book teaches you how to draw and enjoy it even if you feel you have little talent. Useful for stress reduction and self-awareness.

Frankl, Viktor E. *The Unheard Cry for Meaning.* New York: Washington Square Press, 1997.
A book about identity and meaning that can be very useful for women with PMS.

Gendlin, Eugene. *Focusing.* New York: Bantam, 1982.
A technique to identify and change the way your personal problems manifest themselves in your body.

Golub, Sharon, ed. *Lifting the Curse of Menstruation.* New York: Haworth Press, 1983.
Papers reviewing current literature and challenging researchers' assumptions about the role of the menstrual cycle in women's lives.

Hewitt, William H. *Hypnosis for Beginners.* Minneapolis: Llewellyn Publications, 1997.
Explains how to hypnotize yourself and others. Useful section on using hypnosis for relaxation.

Hittleman, Richard. *Yoga: Twenty-Eight-Day Exercise Plan.* New York: Bantam, 1983.

Amply illustrated yoga exercises directed toward relieving many types of physical tension.

————. *Yoga for Health.* New York: Ballantine Books, 1983.
Easy-to-follow instructions for the beginner. Useful nutritional information and recipes; good clear illustrations.

Krieger, Dolores. *The Therapeutic Touch.* New York: Simon and Schuster, 1992.
Clear and concise, this book describes this method of healing and shows how to apply it.

Krimmel, Edward, and Patricia Krimmel. *The Low Blood Sugar Handbook.* Bryn Mawr, PA: Franklin Press, 1992.
A complete book on understanding and managing low blood sugar.

————. *The Low Blood Sugar Cookbook.* Bryn Mawr, PA: Franklin Press, 1992.
Recipes for snacks and complete meals using sugarless, natural foods.

Lark, Susan M. *Dr. Susan Lark's Premenstrual Syndrome Self-Help Book.* Los Angeles: Celestial Arts, 1989.
A self-help approach with diet, exercise, and acupressure massage.

Lauersen, Niels H., and Eileen Stukane. *Premenstrual Syndrome and You.* New York: Simon and Schuster, 1983.
A good beginning book for understanding PMS. Contains a list of PMS resources.

Lee, John R. *What Your Doctor May Not Tell You About Menopause.* New York: Warner, 1996.
Strongly advocates the use of natural, rather than synthetic, hormones in hormone-replacement therapy regimens for perimenopausal and menopausal women.

Madison Pharmacy Associates. *PMS: A Delicate Balance.* Madison, WI: 1993 (by mail order: see page 176).
A thorough and easy-to-read handbook.

Martorano, Joseph. *Unmasking PMS: The Complete Medical Treatment Plan.* New York: M. Evans, 1993.
Includes a simple self-evaluation checklist and describes self-help and prescription treatment options.

McKay, Matthew, Martha Davis, and Beth Eshelman. *The Relaxation and Stress Reduction Workbook.* Oakland, CA: New Harbinger Publications, 1995.
Useful step-by-step techniques for successfully dealing with stress.

Namikoshi, Toru. *The Complete Book of Shiatsu Therapy.* New York: Japan Publications, 1994.
A discussion of principles of Shiatsu therapy and problems it will alleviate.

Nofziger, Margaret. *A Cooperative Method of Natural Birth Control.* Summertown, TN: Book Publishing Company, 1992.
Excellent how-to book for charting ovulation both by basal body temperature and changes in cervical mucus.

Northrup, Christiane. *Women's Bodies, Women's Wisdom.* New York: Bantam, 1998.
Solid guide to connecting physical and emotional health.

Ojeda, Linda. *Exclusively Female.* Claremont, CA: Hunter House, 1983.
Concise information on diet and vitamins for menstrual irregularities, dysmenorrhea, and PMS.

Orbach, Susie. *Fat Is a Feminist Issue II.* New York: Budget Book Service, 1997.
A program for overcoming compulsive eating. Useful to women whose PMS includes loss of control over food.

Reitz, Rosetta. *Menopause: A Positive Approach.* New York: Viking, 1994.
An excellent book about physiological and psychological changes in menopause.

Saunders, Jeraldine, and Harvey M. Ross. *Hypoglycemia: The Classic Health Care Handbook.* New York: Kensington, 1996.

Shaffer, Martin. *Life After Stress.* Chicago: Contemporary Books, 1983.
A good basic book explaining how to assess stress and relieve it.

Somer, Elizabeth. *Nutrition for Women.* New York: Henry Holt, 1993.
Well-documented nutritional guidelines geared toward women's needs.

———. *Food and Mood.* New York: Henry Holt, 1996.

Van Keep, Pieter A., and Wulf H. Utian, eds. *The Premenstrual Syndrome.* Lancaster, Eng.: MTP Press Limited, 1981.
The proceedings of a workshop held during the Sixth International Congress of Obstetrics and Gynecology, Berlin, September 1980. Interesting scientific papers with panel member discussions.

Woolfolk, Robert I., and Frank C. Richardson. *Principles and Practices of Stress Management.* New York: Guilford Press, 1993.
An excellent primer on reducing stress.

Medical Articles

De Lignieres, B., L. Dennerstein, and T. Backstrom. "Influence of Route of Administration on Progesterone Metabolism." *Maturitas* 21 (1995) 251–57.

Gotts, G., L. Dennerstein, and C. A. Morse. "Premenstrual Complaints: An Idiosyncratic Syndrome." *J Psychosom Obstet Gynaecol* 16 (1995) 29–35.

Ellison, P. "Measurement of Salivary Progesterone." *Ann N Y Acad Sci* (1992) 161–76.

Goodale, I. L., A. D. Domar, and H. Benson. "Alleviation of Premenstrual Syndrome Symptoms with the Relaxation Response." *Obstet Gynecol* 75 (1990) 649–55.

Guthrie, J. R., H. G. Burger, J. L. Hopper, and L. Dennerstein. "Hot Flushes, Menstrual Status, and Hormone Levels in a Population-Based Sample of Midlife Women." *Obstet Gynecol* 88 (1996) 437–42.

Hargrove, J. T., W. Maxson, and A. C. Wentz. "Absorption of Oral Progesterone Is Influenced by Vehicle and Particle Size." *American Journal of Obstetrics and Gynecology* 161: (1989) 948–51.

Harlow, S. D., and S. A. Ephross. "Epidemiology of Menstruation and Its Relevance to Women's Health." *Epidemiol Rev* 17 (1995) 265–86.

Kimzey, L. M., J. Fumowski, G. Merriman, G. Grimes, Jr., and L. M. Nelson. "Absorption of Micronized Progesterone from a Nonliquefying Vaginal Cream." *Fertility and Sterility* 56 (1991) 995–96.

Lewis, L. L. "One Year in the Life of a Woman with Premenstrual Syndrome: A Case Study." *Nurs Res* 44 (1995) 111–16.

Lewis, L. L., R. B. Jaffe, J. D. Veldhuis, C. A. Rittenhouse, and E. M. Greenblatt. "Pulsatile Release Patterns of Luteinizing Hormone and Progesterone in Relation to Symptom Onset in Women with Premenstrual Syndrome." *Fertility and Sterility* 64 (1995) 288–92.

Martorano, J. T., M. J. Ahlgrimm, and D. Myers. "Differentiating Between Natural Progesterone and Synthetic Progestogens: Clinical Implications for Premenstrual Syndrome Management." *Comprehensive Therapy* 19 (1993) 96–98.

Maxson, W. S., and J. T. Hargrove. "Bioavailability of Oral Micronized Progesterone." *Fertility and Sterility* 44 (1985) 622–26.

Mortola, J. F., L. Girton, L. Beck, and S. S. Yen. "Diagnosis of Premenstrual Syndrome by a Simple, Prospective, and Reliable Instrument: The calendar of Premenstrual Experiences." *Obstet Gynecol* 76 (1990) 302–7.

Norman, T. R., C. A. Morse, and L. Dennerstein. "Comparative Bioavailability of Orally and Vaginally Administered Progesterone." *Fertility and Sterility* 56 (1991) 1034–39.

Penland, J. G. "Dietary Calcium and Manganese Effects on Menstrual Cycle Symptoms." *Obstet Gynecol* 168 (1993) 1417–23.

Sayegh, R., I. Schiff, J. Wurtman, P. Spiers, J. McDermott, and R. Wurtman. "The Effect of a Carbohydrate-Rich Beverage on Mood, Appetite, and Cognitive Function in Women with Premenstrual Syndrome." *Obstet Gynecol* 86 (1995) 520–28.

Schmidt, P. J., L. K. Nieman, M. A. Danaceau, L. F. Adams, and D. R. Rubinow. "Differential Behavioral Effects of Gonadal Steroids in Women with and in Those Without Premenstrual Syndrome." *New England Journal of Medicine* 338 (1998) 209–16.

Severino, S. K. "Premenstrual Dysphoric Disorder: Controversies Surrounding the Diagnosis." *Harvard Review of Psychiatry* 3 (1996) 293–352.

Severino, S. K., and M. L. Moline. "Premenstrual Syndrome: Identification and Management." *Drugs* 49 (1995) 71–82.

Vanselow, W., B. de Lignieres, K. M. Greenwood, and L. Dennerstein. "Effect of Progesterone and Its 5 Alpha and 5 Beta Metabolites on Symptoms of Premenstrual Syndrome According to Route of Administration." *J Psychosom Obstet Gynaecol* 17 (1996) 29–38.

Vining, R. F., R. A. McGinley, and R. G. Symons. "Hormones in Saliva: Mode of Entry and Consequent Implications for Clinical Interpretation." *Clin Chem* 29/10 (1983) 1752–56.

Vining, R. F., and R. A. McGinley. "The Measurement of Hormones in Saliva: Possibilities and Pitfalls." *J Steroid Biochem* 27 (1987) 81–94.

Resources

PMS

PMS Access
Madison Pharmacy Associates
429 Gammon Place
PO Box 259690
Madison, WI 53719
800-222-4767
www.womenshealth.com

Full Circle Women's Health
1800 30th Street, Suite 308
Boulder, CO 80301
800-418-4040
www.womenshealth@hotmail.com

Natural Hormone Replacement Therapy

Madison Pharmacy Associates
429 Gammon Place
PO Box 259690
Madison, WI 53719
800-558-7046

Endometriosis

Endometriosis Association
8585 N. 76th Place
Milwaukee, WI 53223
800-992-3636

Headaches

American Association for the Study of Headaches
19 Mantua Road
Mt. Royal, NJ 08061
609-423-0043

National Headache Foundation
428 W. St. James Pl., 2nd Floor
Chicago, IL 60614-2750
800-843-2256
www.headaches.org

Hysterectomy

Hysterectomy Educational Resources & Services (HERS)

422 Bryn Mawr Avenue
Bala Cynwyd, PA 19004
610-667-7757

Infertility

Resolve
1310 Broadway Street
Somerville, MA 02144
617-623-0744
www.resolve.org

American Society for Reproductive
    Medicine
1209 Montgomery Highway
Birmingham, AL 35216-2809
205-978-5000
www.asrm.org

Postpartum Depression

Depression After Delivery
P.O. Box 1282
Morrisville, PA 19067
800-944-4773

SYMPTOMS   INITIALS

1. _____ _____

2. _____ _____   Menstruation:

3. _____ _____   Date charting began: _____

MONTHS

1								
2								
3								
4								
5								
6								
7								
8								
9								
10								
11								
12								
13								
14								
15								
16								
17								
18								
19								
20								
21								
22								
23								
24								
25								
26								
27								
28								
29								
30								
31								

Exercise Journal

EXERCISE I LIKE	EXERCISE TO RETRY	EXERCISE I ALWAYS WANTED TO TRY

FIVE EXERCISES TO TRY THIS MONTH

I. Exercise _____ How I will do it _____

_____

_____

2. Exercise _____ How I will do it _____

_____

_____

3. Exercise _____ How I will do it _____

_____

_____

4. Exercise _____ How I will do it _____

_____

_____

5. Exercise _____ How I will do it _____

_____

_____

FILL-IN EXERCISES: While I am trying new forms of exercise I will use the following exercises on a daily basis so that each day I do something.

_____

_____

_____

_____

Weekly Exercise Journal

Use this form to keep track of the exercises you are doing. It will be interesting to see how, over time, your ability and pleasure increase.

Week of _____

	S	M	T	W	T	F	S
EXERCISE							
TIME OF DAY							
HOW LONG							
HOW IT FELT							
WHAT NEEDS TO BE CHANGED							

Bad Day Report

DATE _____ LAST PERIOD _____

DAY OF CYCLE _____

What happened?

Foods eaten (note also any long stretches without eating):

Exercise:

Current stresses:

Review of the day several days later: How does the day look in retrospect? Were issues raised that still may be important? Was your diet that day a healthy one? What have you learned?

INDEX

❁

Page numbers in *italics* refer to charts.

ABOUT THE AUTHORS

———————❈———————

MICHELLE HARRISON, M.D. (www.michelleharrison.com), is a leading authority on women's health and PMS. She developed one of the first programs devoted to treatment of PMS. As a family physician and psychiatrist, she has consulted and lectured internationally om women's health and other related health-policy issues. Dr. Harrison is also the author of *A Woman in Residence* and *The Preteen's First Book About Love, Sex, and AIDS.*

MARLA AHLGRIMM, R.PH., a registered pharmacist, is the cofounder of PMS Access (www.womenshealth.com) and the founder of Women's Health America. She was one of the first health professionals in the United States to recognize, define, and develop PMS options for consumers.

ABOUT THE TYPE

※

This book is set in Garamond, a typeface orginally designed by the Parisian type cutter Claude Garamond (1480–1561). This version of Garamond was modeled on a 1592 specimen sheet from the Egenolff-Berner foundry, which was produced from types assumed to have been brought to Frankfurt by the punch cutter Jacques Sabon (d. 1580).

Claude Garamond's distinguished romans and italics first appeared in *Opera Ciceronis* in 1543–44. The Garamond types are clear, open, and elegant.

SELF-HELP

FOR
PREMENSTRUAL
SYNDROME

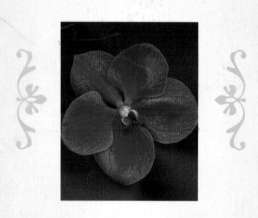

A COMPLETELY REVISED AND UPDATED EDITION
OF THE CLASSIC OF WOMEN'S HEALTH

Third Edition

MICHELLE HARRISON, M.D.,

WITH MARLA AHLGRIMM, R.Ph., FOUNDER OF THE
NATIONAL WOMEN'S HEALTH HOTLINE/PMS ACCESS